D0207867

American Medicine: Challenges for the 1980s

American Medicine: Challenges for the 1980s

David E. Rogers, M.D.

Ballinger Publishing Company • Cambridge, Massachusetts
A Subsidiary of J.B. Lippincott Company

This book is printed on recycled paper.

International Standard Book Number: 0-88410-530-X

Library of Congress Catalog Card Number: 78-16183

Printed in the United States of America

Library of Congress Cataloging in Publication Data

Rogers, David E.
    The changing face of American medicine.

    1. Medical care—United States. 2. Medical centers—United States.
3. Medical education—United States.
I. Title.
RA395.A3R64   362.1'0973   78-16183
ISBN 0-88410-530-X

Contents

List of Figures and Tables

Introduction

Just a decade ago, I moved from being a physician-teacher ministering to *individuals* who came to me for their medical care to a role that required that I think much more carefully about the medical care of *groups* of people, many of whom were unable to find their way into the medical care system. Reasons for this shift in my career were many. I had long been critical about how we handled certain of our affairs in medical academe, an arena in which I had been an enthusiastic participant for twenty-five years. Thus, in part, my career change stemmed from the desire to try to address more directly some of the increasing concerns being voiced about American medicine. In part, too, it stemmed from a belief that one's batteries get recharged by taking on new intellectual and organizational challenges. But perhaps the most compelling reason for the shift was the evidence that many others also felt that the time was ripe to effect constructive change in medicine in America. There was a general national interest apparent in 1968 in improving and strengthening medical care in the United States, and I was captured by the excitement and the potential of participating in this process.

After finishing my formal clinical training in the early 1950s, I had the opportunity to do research during a period when American biomedical research was developing in ways that have revolutionized the way medicine is practiced. As the application of this new biomedical knowledge gained momentum, I participated in expanding the scope of one of the country's medical schools as the chairman of its department of medicine. There I was heavily engaged in the practice of clinical medicine and in teaching young men and women to become doctors. As academic medical centers rethought their roles and their responsibilities on a broader social level during the late 1960s and early 1970s. I helped shape some of these new roles for such a center, as the dean of one of our more prestigious medical schools.

During this professional lifetime, I have seen profound changes in people's attitudes and perceptions about what medicine can or should do. During my early professional career—indeed, for a fifteen year period extending into the early 1960s—medicine could do no wrong. Physicians were highly regarded, and the steady march of new biomedical discoveries led people to high hopes about what medical care could contribute to the quality of American life. These hopes led to the introduction of a flurry of public programs to bring the fruits of biomedical science to all our citizens. Many of the initiatives of the New Frontier and the Great Society were aimed at improving the health and medical care of particular groups of Americans. But as costs began to mount while inequities in care remained, a climate of doubt and concern about the responsiveness of American medicine to perceived needs was increasingly evident. The spectre of a "health care crisis" and the generally sorry state of American medicine were much in the public rhetoric.

During the last five years, we have begun to witness yet another perception about our health care system. This perception has as its central thesis the belief that the one-on-one system of personal physician care actually has very little demonstrable influence on the health status of our society. The argument goes that despite massive increases in medical care costs, we have not seen corresponding benefits in American health; that today's health problems are heavily related to environment and lifestyle and are therefore little influenced by the ministrations of physicians and modern medical technology; and that we should rethink our medically oriented approaches to that better life. Thus a group of critics, ranging from passionate spokesmen like Ivan Illych and Rick Carlson, with their books *Medical Nemesis* and *The End of Medicine*, to physician-historians like Thomas McKeown, or economists like Victor Fuchs, have largely concluded that further investments in our system of individual doctors caring for individual patients should be curtailed in favor of other strategies for improving health. That this theme has gained considerable popularity is indicated by the current national plans for improving health in Canada; by some of the strategies outlined in the forward-planning document for health in the United States that was published last year by the Department of Health, Education, and Welfare; and by a cascading series of programs moving toward self-care, health education, changing lifestyles, and the like.

Thus we are faced at this time with polar views on the role of medicine in society. One group of critics is harsh about the unacceptable costs of American medicine, but at the same time feels that we are not properly applying for the benefit of all what medicine knows how to do. Another set of critics maintains that personal encounter medicine as we know it doesn't make much difference and that we should move away from it to develop other ways of improving the health of Americans.

As with most things, there is significant truth on both sides. That our current system is too expensive is undeniable; but those who wish to have more of what medicine has to offer at lower costs need to have a clearer view of what those costs represent and of the limitations of what medicine can deliver. That it cannot solve all of the ills to which man falls heir or creates for himself is also self-evident, but those who maintain that the personal encounter physician system has failed to improve our people's health should recognize that we are applying the wrong yardsticks if we wish to find out what personal-physician-based medicine actually does. Returning sick people to useful functioning does not show up on the scorecard of death rates from particular disease processes.

During the last six years, I have had a new and expanded view of this scene. It has been a different role—indeed, an experience totally foreign to what I would have predicted when I entered medicine. Developing the programs of The Robert Wood Johnson Foundation and working with trustees, staff, and a whole array of people not ordinarily encountered by doctors who are formulating programs to improve American health and medical care has given me a whole new set of perceptions. Consequently, what I have attempted to do in this book, as even-handedly as I can, is to try to explain several groups of my friends to one another. To lay people concerned about health and national health policy, I would like to try to explain the personal encounter medical system as it exists today—where it seems to be functioning well, what it has accomplished, where its shortfalls lie, and what we can realistically ask of it. I also want them to learn more about the major institutions that create both new knowledge and health professionals and to better understand doctors as people. For my fellow physicians, I would like to point up the areas where our present ways of functioning are found wanting, where we need to rethink our traditional ways of doing things, and where we must join forces with others to distribute more wisely and less expensively the fruits of medicine. As a result, this book is in essence a trilogy. In the first section, I have attempted to describe the status of American medical care today. In it I detail some of the advances we have made during the past decade in bringing more medical care to more

Americans and in improving care for certain special groups. I then turn to my perceptions of where our current system is wanting and where we need to put our emphasis during the next decade if we are to create a more equitable and comprehensive system of medical care for all Americans.

In the second section, I have attempted to look at the institution that creates most of our health professionals—the academic medical center. I do this with the belief that they are one of our more important national institutions, that they are currently under great stress, and that they need both society's understanding and more imaginative leadership to best serve the public that sustains them.

In the last section, I have tried to describe the creature on whom, in the final analysis, the whole system of medicine depends—the physician. Here I offer a very personal view of the kinds of people who elect medical careers; some of the forces, good and bad, that tend to shape them; and some of the problems that confront them in a society that expects a great deal from medicine and medical people.

This, then, is an effort to organize and put to paper my own thoughts about a system of delivering medical care, its major institution, and the professionals within it—subjects that have occupied most of my thoughts and working hours for almost thirty years. In the development of this book, I have had the help and support of a remarkable group of colleagues who have shared in the delightful but demanding task of developing the program and the tone and texture of The Robert Wood Johnson Foundation. They come from rich and varied professional backgrounds in health, business, and the philanthropic world. They include Dr. Walsh McDermott, Dr. Leighton Cluff, Dr. Robert Blendon, Mr. Gustav Lienhard, Miss Margaret Mahoney, Mr. Terrance Keenan, Mr. Frank Karel, and a whole group of young professional colleagues who have helped me take a much more objective and less doctrainaire look at the profession I love and the world in which it operates. Miss Sara Wilkinson has patiently struggled through draft after draft of different parts of the manuscript, and Mrs. Mary Jane Hayes has sleuthed and re-sleuthed some of my vaguer references to be sure that they are accurate. Mrs. Carol Cutler's editing was most helpful in trimming my more discursive rhetoric.

My more humanistic perceptions have been powerfully influenced by my wife, Barbara Lehan Rogers, who has shared in many of my adventures in medicine. Her concern for her fellow humans, her unshakeable belief in their worth, and her wisdom about life has helped mold my own outlook. Her forbearance and her encouragement as this book evolved has been sustaining, and I hope her influence shows in some chapters.

I am basically an optimist by nature. I do not share the cynicism that seems to have so infiltrated the thinking of the day. I like and am excited by change. I have had the privilege of working with remarkable, energetic people throughout my career, and I have watched many of them be or become powerful forces for good. Indeed, popular rhetoric to the contrary, I have seen our medical world change impressively for the better.

So while I have many criticisms about how we do business in medicine today, I have confidence that we can make further progress. My thoughts on how we might go about it will unfold in this volume.

Part I

Medical Care in America: Where Do We Stand Today?

Introduction

About fifteen years ago, this nation set about putting right all of the things that were troubling us about medical care. We were at that time in a confident and vigorous national mood. During the two decades that followed World War II, the United States made a remarkable commitment to improving medical care for all its citizens, a comment that reached full flower during the early 1960s. This was but part of a broad agenda that derived from a general optimism about our collective abilities to better shape our society. During that period, Americans had high hopes—indeed, considerable confidence—that we could fashion our society to offer more equity and a higher quality of life to all who lived in the United States. Thus, we were putting substantial amounts of our public funds to work on our social problems. The cheerful belief prevailed that, given the proper resources, professionals and laymen in the public and private sectors, working cooperatively together, could produce dramatic improvements in the texture and meaning of the lives of all Americans.

This optimism seemed to rest on solid footing. Our successes with the space program, the victory over poliomyelitis, the expanding economy, and a growing respect for the splendid technologic base that had been developed in American medicine all fanned the feeling that money plus technology plus human effort could produce a better life for our citizens at reasonable costs. These were gloriously idealistic times in which we were determined to eliminate poverty, abolish racial discrimination, do away with substandard housing, revitalize our cities, and provide first class educational opportunities and good medical care for all. In all of these sectors, many were busily working to remedy problems.

The public agenda in matters medical seemed relatively straight-forward. First and foremost, Americans were deeply concerned about the rapidly escalating costs of medical care. Indeed it was primarily costs that were responsible for mounting criticisms of virtually all areas of the medical care system. For a number of years, consumer costs of hospital care had risen at rates twice those of other commodities, and these costs seemed unreasonably and inequitably distributed. Lay magazines had tragic stories to tell about individuals and families who were financially ruined by a single major illness, and even the cost of basic office and clinic visits presented a serious roadblock to medical care for many with marginal incomes. Perhaps most troubling was an uneasy feeling that despite these enormous flows of money, medical care was getting worse. The term "health care crisis" was much heard in the discussions of the day.

The second general area of concern was the increasing difficulty Americans were having in obtaining ambulatory care—the kind of out-of-hospital care most of us need most of the time. This difficulty was experienced by rich, poor, and middle income people alike. Too few health resources existed in rural and urban poverty areas, and too many people, particularly those who were poor or black or elderly or isolated, lacked ready access to appropriate services. Doctors and other health professionals who rendered general medical care seemed to be increasingly hard to find. The country was concerned about the lack of adequate numbers of doctors, and there were just not enough physicians and their associates who were willing and able to handle first contact medicine or preventive care; nor was there any structure to sustain health professionals in these areas. Furthermore, the distribution of physicians and associated personnel by medical specialty seemed increasingly out of line with needs: There was clearly a shortage of those who delivered primary or general care and increasing evidence of a mounting oversupply of physicians in certain specialty areas.

Last of the concerns about medical care in the 1960s was a general uneasiness about the loss of human caring—the "samaritan" functions of medicine. Many people felt that physicians and other health personnel lacked interest and/or skill in understanding and coping with the anxiety, despair, and loneliness that often accompany illness. While it was generally agreed that we had developed a system that could deliver sophisticated and complex medical care in situations of life-threatening illness, medicine was found to be wanting in bringing appropriate and compassionate understanding and personal support to those seeking medical care.

This then was the agenda of the midsixties, and many programs and significant resources were being directed toward addressing these problems. Public insurance in the form of Medicare and Medicaid had been enacted to offset the personal costs of medical care for certain groups. Neighborhood health centers were being built. Federal legislation was enacted to provide care for mothers, infants and poor children, and programs were established in many cities to carry it out. Centers for the study and treatment of mental retardation and mental illness were rising in a number of cities. An enormous number of public dollars were being poured into efforts to bring the fruits of American biomedical science to all of our citizens and to correct many of the inequities and shortfalls that had been identified. Many programs of the New Frontier and the Great Society were directed at bringing more services to people.

However, by the late 1960s and escalating steadily into the early 1970s, the climate of optimism began to change. By this time, the fact that we had not been able to swiftly and simply accomplish the laudable social goals we had set for ourselves in medicine and elsewhere was readily evident. A sense of increasing frustration and disillusionment began to pervade the national scene. These failures troubled us and rested heavily on the American conscience. In the despair caused by these failures, blame was freely distributed in all directions, and there was increasingly bitter rhetoric and often tragic strife between various groups who had previously shared many of the same goals. Thus by the early 1970s, we had a paradox of a country enjoying continuing economic growth and a high level of scientific achievement that was tormented by doubts about its abilities for self-renewal and was generally quite uncertain about its capacities to marshal its resources to meet the problems of those in need. The discouraged included not only those who believed in a central attack on social problems but also those who did not. Consequently, many felt that our nation's resources had been misdirected in our efforts to correct social inequities, that these vexing conditions could not be solved rationally through social programs, and that they did not deserve the priorities or the funds that had been assigned to them. A general cynical attitude that any attempt to change things in the system generally made them worse seemed to prevail. That we were simply "throwing money at social problems" was the popular parlor comment of the day, and the feeling that a self-governing society such as ours was unable to cope with these kinds of problems became increasingly common.

Since the dashing of the high hopes of the midsixties, we have passed through a progressively more troubled decade. It has been one of our most intense periods of self-doubt, self-examination, and change in social attitudes. Many of our traditional ways of doing and thinking about things have been challenged, and changes that would have been unheard of in decades past have been taking place. It has been a period of wrenching disillusionment and disbelief, as we have watched the accelerating disintegration of our inner cities, continuing racial tensions, a terrifying increase in crimes of violence, and the shocking erosion of American morality in high places; epitomized by the Watergate scandal. Despite the final abandonment of an unpopular war, we have plunged from a vigorous and productive economy into the greatest economic recession since the Great Depression of the 1930s, and we are now struggling with the paradox of worrisome inflation coupled with high rates of unemployment. Most recently, we have been confronted with the disquieting realization that we are running out of many resources we previously believed to be infinite.

Thus, in one short decade we have seen a striking change in national attitudes. We have moved from high optimism about our capacity to change our world to general discouragement and cynicism about our individual and institutional abilities to cope with the social problems of our modern society. We seem to have lost much of our traditional "can do" American enthusiasm.

Through this decade has also run the conviction that things have also grown steadily worse in medicine. Despite the efforts to improve medical care that I have cited, the continuing rise in costs has been accompanied by a general feeling that the medical care system is failing badly. Maldistribution of services, bad management of medical care institutions, and the poor quality of care administered to many of those less fortunate than others has been much discussed in speeches, articles, and television programs. Americans are deeply worried about the specter of serious illness and the ability of the medical care system to cope with it effectively and affordably. A recent newspaper article gave an interesting peek at this private world of individual worry. In a report of what people pray about, medical matters led the list. Of 71,000 requests for prayers sent to a particular religious organization, almost 50 percent ranked serious illness and other health matters as most troubling.[1]

This change in attitudes about our collective abilities to advance and improve our society troubles me. It runs the hazard of being self-fulfilling. The fact that the kinds of social issues we have attempted to attack do not lend themselves to conventional or short-term economic or political responses does not necessarily mean they are insoluable. These are complex problems that require real understanding of their origins, plenty of time, great patience, a willingness to undergo some individual sacrifices for the common good, and the cooperative efforts of many to move in appropriate directions.

I have a more optimistic view of what has transpired during the last decade. During the past two years, the foundation with which I am associated has made a rather careful survey of available evidence to determine just what actually has happened in the field of medical care and to the health of Americans during this generally dishearten-ing period.[2] The results are both surprising and encouraging. The evidence—and it is unequivocal—suggests that we have improved our ways of delivering medical care to those who need it. In certain sectors, the changes for the better are impressive. In our peculiarly American way, many individual groups, and institutions, have con-tributed to the strengthening of medical care services in this country, but many of these changes have gone almost unrecognized, even by those who have done the most to effect the improvement. True, we have not gone as far as I would have wished—social change seems to take much too long—and there are many equally complex and con-tentious problems remaining that need attention. But the fact that we have made real progress in some very difficult areas relating to medical care suggests that we can do likewise in those areas that re-main problems. Although it is a large task that cannot be accom-plished without enormous cooperative efforts on the parts of many, I am persuaded that we have the human resources and talents to solve the problems that remain if several conditions are met. First, we need to be once again unembarrassed about striving for appar-ently simplistic goals like equality in access to medical care, or proper care for our children, or more considerate treatment of our elderly. Second, we must regain our confidence that we have the capacity within us and our social institutions to make the appro-priate changes in our system and not let the cynics deflect us. Third, we must precisely and objectively isolate and identify the shortfalls and problems and then accurately target our efforts to correct them. Last, we need to develop a more realistic view of the time necessary to accomplish our objectives. One of the compelling lessons to be learned from the changes made in the last decade is that they took time, continuing attention, and singleness of purpose—but so do most things that are lasting and worthwhile.

Part I of this book is an effort to tote up the scorecard—to point out where we have already made progess and what remains as an agenda for the future. It is my hope that reviewing how far we have come and where we still must go can help move us from our un-warranted national pessimism regarding past effort to improve health and medical care, for such an attitude subtel blocks progress. We need a more optimistic frame of mind if we are to move more swiftly, and I think we can. Five years ago I stated my conviction that "by the conscious and voluntary actions of people, it is possible to better the human condition."[3] The evidence of progress made during the last decade reinforces that belief. That we have not done it all will be readily evident, but we have made a start.

✳ *Chapter 1*

The Development of
Medicine in America

To understand the central problems in medical care that concerned Americans a decade ago, it is helpful to understand some of the history of American medicine as it has evolved in this nation, for it differs quite sharply from that on the European continent from which we sprang. In Colonial times, many lay people were involved in medical affairs. While in England and on the Continent medicine was well established and professionally controlled, we did not import it to this country. Those initially settling this nation wished to cast off the rigid social caste system that characterized British society of that day, and medicine was part of that system. A humorous remark made in 1728 by William Byrd, a distinguished resident of Colonial Virginia, captures the feeling of those times. In explaining why America had appealed to many, he stated that it stemmed from the fact that "it was a place free from those three great scourges of mankind—priests, lawyers, and physicians."[1]

THE AMERICAN PHYSICIAN

The American physician emerged in a highly informal fashion. He did everything from shaving beards to mixing drugs to performing major surgery, and he had neither legal nor professional constraints. Although some universities had established units for training doctors by the middle of the eighteenth century, in the main it was privately owned profit-making proprietary medical schools that shaped American medicine through most of the nineteenth century. By the late 1800s, we had 450 medical schools—almost four times the present

number—and virtually all of them were proprietary.[2] The only requirements for admission were the money to pay the tuition and the
ability to read and write. These schools were shockingly bad by
modern standards, but, in retrospect, perhaps they suited the needs
of the times better than might be thought. They trained large
numbers of physicians; there were many more physicians per capita
than there are now. The cost of both medical education and medical
care was low, and physicians were in sufficient supply, so that almost
no small town was without its general practitioner. Bear in mind that
at that time there was very little in the way of a scientific base for
medicine. Most remedies were based on dogma and tradition, and
there was little that medicine could actually do in the way of meaningful disease intervention. Thus the lack of an education that we
would deem appropriate for a physician today probably did not
make too much difference.

But by the turn of the century, there were increasing concerns
about the low standards—indeed, the *absence* of standards—in medical practice of the day. Specialists were coming onto the scene, many
of them trained in Europe, who were very critical of the proprietary
medical schools. University medical schools were beginning to be
developed; the Johns Hopkins University launched a medical institution based on European models with a strong laboratory and science
base. In this setting—in part prodded by the concerns of the newly
formed American Medical Association, which was at that time a
force for medical reform—a nonphysician, Abraham Flexner, published a report in 1910 that was a scathing comentary on the medical
education system.[3] This report pulled no punches. Flexner was
vitriolic in his comments about proprietary medical schools, recom-
mending that they all be closed. He indicated that medical education
was a sham, lacking educational standards, supervision, and goals. He
came out strongly for giving medical education a university base
grounded in science and for developing a competent faculty whose
primary responsibility was that of educating future physicians.

Flexner's report produced dramatic changes in medical education.
The proprietary medical diploma mills were eliminated, better
curricula were structured in those schools that remained, laws for
licensing physicians were established, and in a fairly short period,
medicine moved from an apprenticeship art to a genuinely professional education, increasingly founded on science.

The system of medical practice established at that time was based
on the premise that each family should have a responsible physician,
that the majority of doctors would be general practitioners giving
care to their constituents, and that a small cadre of specialists would

offer consultation and special services to those rendering general care. This system served us well through the first part of this century. However, a series of events starting in the early 1920s has changed this picture quite dramatically. Beginning with the discovery of insulin in 1922 and proceeding through the development of the sulfanimides, antibiotics, and other potent drugs for the management of anemia, hypertension, cardiac failure malignancies, and the like, the march of science-based medicine has continued at an accelerating pace, greatly expanding the armamentarium of medicine. These changes placed an increasing number of remarkable new tools and therapies in the hands of the personal physician, which meant that he could actually modify or even cure an impressive number of human illnesses. The increasing use of anesthesia, the introduction of better surgical techniques, the protection offered by antimicrobials, and the development of synthetic substances that permit the replacement or introduction of tubes or pins or joints into the human body have also vastly increased the capabilities of the modern physician.

And herein lay part of the dilemma. To use these tools precisely and appropriately required new knowledge and new skills. No longer could the "all purpose" physician command sufficient knowledge to deal with all the ills of his patients; thus, the march toward specialization began. Pressures for specialization also came from patients. As the public became more and more aware of what medicine could offer, consumers of medical care, particularly upper and middle class people in metropolitan areas, began to insist on consultation and care by physicians with specialist labels. Specialists steadily gained in status and were able to command much higher fees. Given that specialization meant higher status and more money and more control over one's time, the march of physicians in this direction was inevitable. Academic medical centers were increasingly staffed by full-time, fully salaried physicians who were themselves specialists, and they largely replaced those of generalist orientation as teachers. Thus those who practiced general medicine, those who handled most of the continuing care of people with out of hospital needs, came primarily to be the dropouts from postdoctoral training; internists, surgeons, pediatricians, obstetrician-gynecologists, psychiatrists, and an increasing number of other medical and surgical specialists became the order of the day.

THE DEVELOPMENT OF THE AMERICAN HOSPITAL

Occurring parallel with the trend toward specialization and complementing the development of new technologies that could be applied by medicine came the emergence of the modern hospital. During the early days of our nation, hospitals were in relatively small demand. They were developed largely for the sick poor and the incurable, and most of the care given therein was nursing care. Indeed, it was not until late in the nineteenth century that hospitals could accurately be said to benefit patients. Following her stint as a nurse in the Crimean War, Florence Nightingale wrote that "the very first requirement in the hospital is that it should do the sick no harm";[4] In the 1850s at the time of her writing, this was often in doubt.

The increasing urbanization of America was a powerful stimulus for the evolving American hospital. The congregation of people in the cities concentrated the need for medical care. This need, coupled with the medical profession's requirements for teaching and research facilities, led to the founding of an increasing number of voluntary urban hospitals. Thus, while in 1876 there were fewer than 200 hospitals in the nation, by the 1950s this number had expanded to 6,788—a growth of almost 200 hospitals per year.[5] Hospitals also underwent a dramatic transformation in their character and complexity. Many of the rapidly expanding medical technologies could be based only in a hospital, and the increasing utilization of physicians by a steadily expanding population, coupled with a decreasing use of house calls to manage illness, pushed physicians and hospitals more closely together.

The advances in the last seventy-five years have thus profoundly changed the character of medical practice, the kinds of doctors who work in it, and its major place of business. The technologic changes that gave new tools to the personal physician, coupled with public health achievements in improving environmental sanitation, controlling insect vectors, developing clean water and clean food supplies, and immunizing the population against a number of plagues of the past, have led to a remarkable change in the kinds of diseases to which we fall heir and have dramatically improved an individual's chance of survivng to adulthood. Mortality rates for children between the ages of one and four are now less than one-tenth of what they were in 1920, and there has been a dramatic shift in the kinds of diseases and problems causing childhood deaths. Whereas influenza, pneumonia, diarrhea, and diptheria led the list in the 1920s, killing 988 children per 100,000 in this age group, accidents and congenital defects top the list today, killing fewer than 84 per 100,000.[6] The fact that most children born healthy can survive to adulthood has also played a role in changing attitudes regarding family size and indirectly, toward mean family income. The elimination of many other plagues of the past—typhoid fever, typhus, smallpox, and poliomyelitis—and the development of drugs that permit the effective treatment of tuberculosis, syphilis, pneumonia, puerperal fever, meningococcal meningitis, and certain other illnesses have also profoundly changed the character of American life.

But while certain diseases have been eliminated, others remain or have become more prevalent. As our population comes to contain more and more older people, problems of coronary artery disease, cancer, chronic lung disease, diabetes, crippling forms of arthritis, and the like have loomed as leading causes of disability and death. We have worked intensely to identify the causes and to find cures for these diseases, but to date they continue to elude us. We have much tougher nuts to crack today then we formerly did, and the technologies employed in treating these diseases have grown complex and costly. This technologic sophistication, which can modify but not cure disease, has become a two-edged sword—at times life-saving, but at the same time a major cause of the rising costs of medical care.

EFFORTS TO OFFSET THE COSTS OF MEDICAL CARE

Over 40 years ago to offset individual costs of these increasingly expensive diseases and to provide a more stable base for our hospitals and our medical technology, we began to develop third-party mechanisms for paying for medical care. The establishment of Blue Cross in the 1930s, the entry of other private insurance carriers onto the scene, and the enactment of public insurance programs, Medicare and Medicaid, during the 1960s have all been efforts to address this problem. Thus in 1976, over 93 percent of Americans had some form of health insurance.[7] That insurance coverage is too incomplete, that hardships continue to fall on those least able to pay, that families can still be financially wiped out by catastrophic illness, and that health insurance has been inflationary are all true. However, we have attempted to move, albeit in fumbling fashion, to protect people against unmanageable medical care costs that in great measure have resulted from improvements in medical care. Paradoxically, in attempting to finance the costs of medical care, we stopped short of making the changes in financing mechanisms that might have helped put a brake on these costs. Because of the unexpected expenses of Medicare and Medicaid, we did not move to finance ambulatory care—a less expensive way of delivering services—and we did not make provisions to protect against the costs of catastrophic illness.

These, then, were some of the forces that led to the situation in which we found ourselves a decade ago. Medical science had developed increasing knowledge about human illness and how to deal with it, making the proper application of medical skills more important and more demanding. This in turn led to changes in the nature of the education of physicians and to marked increases in its costs. An increasing number of physicians specialized to be able to use those tools most effectively. Hospitals, initially institutions for nursing care for the incurable and the sick poor, became an increasingly important place for delivering care as America moved from an agrarian society to a highly urbanized, industrialized nation. More and more doctors moved to the hospital to make use of the technologies available to them there. While all this was happening, the patterns of disease that characterized our society changed remarkably. But changing disease patterns have not meant the absence of illness, and the problem of an increasing number of people with complex, long-term chronic illness remains, along with the need for increasingly expensive technologies to deal with them. In an effort to cope with expenses, we developed insurance systems to reduce the financial burdens of illness of the individual, and these in turn helped escalate the costs of medical care. The solution of certain problems had brought yet others: an alarming escalation of medical care costs; insufficient numbers of primary care physicians and ambulatory care facilities; marked inequities in access to and the quality of care received by certain groups; and an unappealing impersonality in the delivery of care.

Chapter 2

Changes in Medical Care and Health, 1966–1976

To grapple with the problems that troubled Americans in the late 1950s and during the 1960s, we put large amounts of money and a vast array of new programs to work. When viewed in the late 1960s, the results of these efforts seemed discouraging. How do things look a decade later? Have the programs that were initiated during the sixties accomplished anything?

PHYSICIAN CARE

Is physician care as difficult to come by as it was a decade ago? The answer is no; people seem to be seeing doctors more frequently. While data on the number of visits people make to doctors do not tell us all that we wish to know, because they do not tell us what went on during the encounter, they do offer one index of how medical services are deployed. They are markedly improved. Between 1966 and 1976, physician visits per person per year rose by 19 percent.[1] This suggests that physicians are more accessible. Even more encouraging are the indications that physician care is now more available to those who need it most. Of principal concern a decade ago were the marked inequities in the availability of care for those who were poor or near poor. In the 1930s, people of low income saw a physician only about one-half as often as those with higher incomes, an inequality compounded by the fact that serious illness is more common among the poor. By the mid-1960s, this gap had been reduced, but people with low incomes still saw physicians 16 percent less frequently than did those of high income. By 1975, however, this inequity in the availability of physician services had been largely eliminated. Taken collectively, people of low income are now seeing physicians slightly more often than those of high income, averaging six visits per year compared to a national average of about five.[2] This suggests that we have found ways of getting low income people into the health system and at a frequency that is more commensurate with their larger numbers of health problems. That these figures can be applied fairly broadly is also suggested by the sharp decrease in the numbers of Americans not seeing a physician at all during a particular year. In 1966, 32 percent of Americans fell in this category. This had dropped to 25 percent by 1976.[3] During the same decade, there was also improvement in the availability of physicians to minority groups. In 1966, black Americans saw physicians 31 percent less often than did white Americans. By 1976 this gap had largely disappeared. Blacks, also a group with greater burdens of illness, were as a group seeing physicians nearly as frequently as whites. These improvements in patient access to a doctor's care have been significantly assisted by the rapid growth of both private and public health insurance coverage. Since 1960, the proportion of the patient's bill paid out of pocket has been reduced by 40 percent.[4]

Gratifying though these figures are, they need to be interpreted with great caution. Obviously if one believes, as I do, that better medical care can improve the health and welfare of Americans, getting to medical care is a prerequisite for all that follows. But there is evidence that some of the medical care being given to previously undercared for groups is not all that it should be. Scandalous Medicaid "mills" and overcrowded hospital emergency rooms and out-patient departments are the sites of much of this new care. Further, there is considerable evidence that some of the visits are to inappropriate sources of care—patients with chronic problems overwhelming the resources of acute care facilities and some patients with problems that could be handled on an ambulatory basis end up in hospitals beds. Thus, we need much better evidence that a physician visit yields appropriate medical care than the above figures can tell us. The point remains, however, that our effort to improve access to care have resulted in change and that it seems to be change in the proper direction.

NUMBERS OF HEALTH PROFESSIONALS

What of the crisis in the production of health professionals? In the midsixties, much criticism was leveled at academic institutions because they had not increased the number of young men and women being trained as doctors, dentists, nurses, and other health professionals. In contrast to the foregoing statistics on patient visits, where the data are admittedly soft, here the changes are inarguable. Between 1966 and 1976, medical school increased the number of physicians in training by more than 70 percent. While only slightly more than 34,000 young men and women were in American medical schools in 1966, almost 60,000 were in training in 1976.[5]

Also of deep concern in the midsixties was the homogeneity of those being admitted to medical school. Medical students were overwhelmingly white, male, and from middle and upper income backgrounds. That this did not well serve our racially and culturally heterogeneous nation was self-evident, and efforts to increase the numbers of women, blacks, Spanish-speaking Americans, and American Indians in medical school were initiated. Here we have also made progress. Whereas only 8 percent of entering students in 1966 were women, this had risen to nearly 25 percent in 1976. While only a shocking 2.5 percent of entering medical students were from black and other minority backgrounds in 1966, this had risen to about 9 percent in 1976.[6] That this change in the mix of entering students has come too slowly and too unevenly, with only a small number of institutions leading the way, is undeniable. Nevertheless, change has occurred, and it is change in the proper direction.

At the same time, more opportunities for physicians in training to pursue generalist careers are being developed in an effort to redress the specialist-generalist imbalance. Residency opportunities for those interested in generalist careers are rapidly expanding, and American-trained physicians are filling most of these.

Nursing schools have also increased their enrollments by an impressive 90 percent,[7] and the clinical training of nurse graduates has been broadened and strengthened to give them greater and more direct patient care responsibilities. The number of people enrolling in dental school in 1976 was almost 50 percent higher than in 1966 and, as in medical schools, an increasing proportion are women or minority group members.[8] A number of dental schools are training their graduates to serve groups of people with special dental care needs, notably the physically and mentally handicapped. As another sign of progress, new kinds of health workers are entering the field in rapidly increasing numbers. The physician assistant, for example, was virtually nonexistent in 1966. Programs to train these new health professionals have now been developed in more than fifty-five institutions, and more than 2,000 young men and women enrolled in these programs in 1976.[9]

These changes in the nature and number of health professionals suggest institutional responsiveness of a high order. Indeed, there are some indications that we may be overshooting projected national needs for trained health manpower.

CARE FOR SPECIAL GROUPS WITH SPECIAL PROBLEMS

The past decade has also seen some rather convincing demonstrations that the organization of medical care for special groups with special problems can substantially reduce hospital costs, mortality, and the burdens of chronic illness. All of these programs were initiated because massive infusions of federal funds were directed toward improving medical care for the needy. To cite three examples:

Improving Care for Expectant Mothers and Their Offspring

First, the introduction of maternal and infant care programs to provide better medical care to low income groups, which were initiated during the 1960s and early 1970s, was paralleled by an overall reduction in neonatal deaths from 20 to 15.5 per 1,000 live births among the predominantly black high-risk population served by these special programs. This represented an impressive 23 percent decline in infant mortality in this group over a five year period.[10] The results from several cities served to dramatize these results. In Denver, following the institution of the program, there was a fall in infant mortality from 34.2 per 1,000 live births in 1964 to 21.5 per 1,000 live births in 1969 in the twenty-five census tracts in which mothers were offered these services. In Birmingham, Alabama, there was a decrease in the infant death rate from 24.5 to 14.3 during the same time period. One of the most dramatic results was documented in Omaha, Nebraska. Here, the maternal and infant care program resulted in the reduction in infant deaths from 33.4 per 1,000 live births in 1964 to 13.4 in 1969—a 60 percent decline in infant wastage in those who were enrolled in the program.[11] These are genuinely remarkable achievements. While one cannot directly attribute these reductions in mortality to the introduction of better care—many other changes were occurring simultaneously—they suggest that this program introduced in the sixties, which was generally considered a relative failure, did indeed have an impact on precisely the problem at which it was directed.

That such care need not be complex or expensive is suggested by data from the Frontier Nursing Service in Kentucky. This institution succeeded in reducing infant death rates by 64 percent in a poverty-stricken rural area through an organized system of nurse and midwife care.[12] A similar result was obtained in Georgia, where the introduction of a maternal and infant care program sharply reduced prematurity and lowered infant mortality by 40 percent in the counties served, as compared to similar adjacent counties in which no such services were available.[13]

Improving Care for Children

Federally financed medical care programs designed for low income children provide a second graphic example of this point. Here again, the evidence seems solid that health services can be improved and can yield financial savings at the same time. For example, the number of days of hospitalization per 1,000 children registered in these federally financed youth clinics dropped from 101 at the inception of the program in 1968 to 42 in 1972. Of further importance, the annual cost per registrant fell from $201 to $131 during the same period.[14] Carefully studied individual programs caring for youngsters in the Boston Pediatric Center and in a neighborhood center in Rochester, New York, yielded similar results. The Boston Pediatric Center reduced the need for hospitalization of children by 36 percent in just two years following the introduction of their comprehensive program.[15] In Rochester, the results were a 50 percent reduction in the number of hospital days required for children participating in the project.[16] In both instances, the amount of time children were ill or out of school was also dramatically reduced. A study of a comprehensive health program for children in a poor section of East Baltimore showed a 60 percent reduction in the incidence of rheumatic fever in children enrolled in the program. Translated into human terms, in the five years prior to the introduction of the program, rheumatic fever, with its significant aftermath of crippling heart disease, developed in fifty-one children in the target area. Only eleven in the same area were so afflicted during a similar period while receiving well-organized care. This means that forty children were spared possible heart disease of a kind that used to kill many in young adulthood.[17]

Improving Care for Those With Certain Chronic Illnesses

Chronic illness is a third area where specially designed medical care has been shown to make a heartening difference. An impressive study in Memphis—a joint effort of the local health department, the Memphis Hospital, and the University of Tennessee—showed that a staff of specially trained nurses, placed in decentralized and accessible facilities and guided by protocols, could profoundly reduce the cost of ambulatory care for diabetic patients. Over a two year period, the cost of this care was reduced to one-fifth of the cost of care given to diabetics in the medical center. At the same time, there was a 42 percent reduction in hospitalization required for these diabetic patients.[18] Similar encouraging results have been obtained in managing patients with hypertension in less costly workplace settings in New York City and in improving the care of patients with chronic pulmonary disease in a similar kind of program on the California coast. All of these studies suggest that there are ways of managing special groups and special problems much more satisfactorily than in times past—and at costs that we can afford.

THE IMPROVING HEALTH OF AMERICANS

There are also some significant indications that the health of Americans has improved over this last decade. By no means am I suggesting that this is a direct result of improving access to care or of better application of medical services to those who need them. Indeed, there has been no evidence at all that I am aware of that the improved health of Americans is the result of more medical care. Nevertheless, the following data do seem to indicate that we are not going down the road to ruin.[19]

First, death rates of Americans have been falling for the last ten years. Between the mid-1950s and the late 1960s, age-adjusted death rates were fairly constant or fell only slightly. During the last eight years, however, they have dropped by almost 14 percent. This rate of decrease is as high as we have seen anytime during this century. Calculated on a population base of 100,000, the death rate stood at 746.7 in 1968, but had dropped to 642.1 in 1975. Similarly, infant mortality rates have continued to decline, again without much heralding. Between 1960 and 1976, they fell by 42 percent, from 26 to 15.1 infant deaths per thousand live births, the lowest ever recorded in the United States, and infant mortality rates are continuing to decline. This is of particular interest because the conventional wisdom of roughly a decade ago was that we had then gone about as far as we could go toward reducing neonatal death rates. While family planning activities are an important component of this change, they do not constitute the whole story. The decrease in infant mortality has been accompanied by an impressive drop in maternal mortality. Between 1960 and 1976, maternal mortality dropped by 61 percent, from 37 to 14.5 deaths per 100,000 live births. We should not become too complacent about these reduced infant and maternal mortality rates—similar improvements have occurred in most of the industrialized Western nations—but it is change in an appropriate direction.

There are still other indicators of improving health in the United States. The story of coronary heart disease, our number one killer, is a fascinating illustration. After the initial recognition of coronary artery disease in 1912, deaths reported from it increased steadily through the 1930s, 1940s, and 1950s. While it is generally believed that this increase has continued relentlessly, in fact, the age-adjusted death rates due to coronary artery disease peaked in 1963, although this was not well recognized until ten years later. During the twelve year period between 1963 and 1976, death rates ascribed to coronary artery disease have fallen by 23 percent. Indeed, during the seven years from 1968 to 1975, they fell by 18 percent. Thus, not only is a drop occurring, it seems to be accelerating. Although this is quite a dramatic change, the reasons for the decrease are not known. Is it more exercise, less consumption of saturated fats, the declining use of cigarettes, less stress, better medical treatment, or a combination of these? That we do not know the reasons for this change is frustrating, but it does not alter the fact. As a matter of fact, eleven of the first fifteen causes of death in the United States have declined during this period. This includes death due to strokes, diabetes, peptic ulcers, and a number of other disease problems. Only deaths due to cancer, cirrhosis, and suicide and homicide have shown increases.[20]

These are the encouraging signs of progress. We have in place a technically sophisticated medical care system that is well equipped to handle the most acute kinds of life-threatening illnesses. We have a generous number of hospitals, reasonably distributed, most giving quite respectable care to those admitted to them. We now have adequate numbers of well-trained health professionals, an increasing number of whom are women and minority groups members, to take care of our medical needs. We have broadened our ways of financing care, particularly for those most in need, although we have paid dearly for it. We have improved access to care for many Americans, most notably for those most poorly served ten years ago—those who are black or poor or both. We have clearly demonstrated that we can develop systems to further reduce infant and maternal mortality and to give more effective care to children. We have some programs in place that show we can do a better job, at affordable costs, with certain kinds of chronic disease problems. In addition, certain gross indicators of the health of Americans, how many die and of what, have also improved.

These are encouraging evidences of progress. They suggest that our efforts of a decade ago were not misdirected, that we can, albeit slowly, move in socially appropriate directions. These data should give us confidence for approaching those problems that remain. I believe that they also illustrate another point: They show how subtly change can occur over a long period of time without our recognizing it has taken place. There is a characteristic cycle in our impatient American approach to social problems. First there is long period of increasing concern, turbulence, and mounting awareness of the serious nature of a defect in the system. This is often followed by a brief, frantic period of rhetoric, legislation, funding, and a much-publicized commitment to correct the problem overnight. This is followed in turn by a short period of intense activity with little apparent effect. Alas, there usually follows a period of discouragement and disenchantment—a general feeling that we are on the wrong track. Public attention wanes, and any continued efforts are derided as another example of "do-gooder" ineptitude. A period passes; then, all of a sudden, changes for the better appear to take place almost overnight. We are surprised and pleased by this, but often forget what went before. We need a better institutional memory, a greater willingness to stay with programs, and a longer, more realistic perspective on such matters. We have made significant progress in correcting certain problems in medical care perceived as important to Americans ten years ago. What is needed now is a precise characterization of the problems that remain, clear assessment of those particular problems, and "having at them."

※ *Chapter 3*

The Remaining Agenda—
Where Are the Shortfalls?

Broadly speaking, there are two major problems in medical
care that should serve as our agenda for the future. First,
the costs of medical care are rising too rapidly, and we
must find ways of containing them. Second, while we have made encouraging progress in improving access to medical care for most
Americans during the last decade, there are some special groups to
which we should now direct our attention. Four groups of Americans—poor children, poor elderly, rural dwellers, and the handicapped—each hampered by dependency or isolation, continue to
have problems in getting their appropriate share of medical services.
One other group, people with chronic long-term illnesses, is not
getting full benefit from what we now know how to do to improve
their functioning and comfort.

THE UNACCEPTABLE COSTS OF MEDICAL CARE

The central problem that has led to such an intense focus on American medicine—that of costs—remains very much with us. Indeed, it
has become yet more serious. Anxieties about cost tend to obscure
or keep us from attacking other problems in medical care. Unless we
can satisfactorily contain and properly distribute costs, we will
simply not get at any of the second order problems which I believe
are equally compelling. There are two parts to the cost problem.
First, they are unacceptably high; second, despite our expenditures,
there are still too many Americans left out of coverage for medical
care.

In 1976, Americans spent an average of $552 per person, or almost

$2,300 per family, on health and medical care. This contrasts dramatically with the $180 per person Americans spent just a decade ago. Total health care expenditures in the United States now consume almost $150 billion, or close to 9 percent of the gross national product. Hospital care now costs ten times more per capita than it did in 1950, and four times as much as it did in 1966.[1] For the average American, health care expenditures now consume between 7.5 and 10 percent of personal income.[2] During the past six years, health care costs have risen an average of $10 billion yearly, and all agree that the present rate of increase—more than two times that of the consumer price index—simply cannot continue.[3]

Numbers in billions lack meaning for most of us, so let me make these statistics somewhat more graphic. During the last twenty-four hours, the rise in cost of care for Americans—not the total cost, just the increase—was more than $30 million. If you sat down to read this book an hour ago, medical and health care costs have increased by $1.25 million since you put your eyes to paper. This is alarming to even the most enthusiastic advocates of full medical care services for all.

The other part of the cost problem relates to our continuing failure to distribute services effectively and appropriately. Despite the massive infusion of new dollars, there are still too many people not covered adequately or at all by either private or public programs. In the United States today there are approximately thirty-four million people, largely the poor and near poor, who are basically unable to pay for their medical care.[4] Because of the way the Medicaid program was designed, approximately one-fourth of these thirty-four million low income people are not covered by any public insurance program at all.[5] Although considered a program for the poor at large, Medicaid is actually a program for those on welfare. This is a group synonymous with the poor in popular imagination, but not in reality. It is also a fact that most moderate income people still do not have significant out of hospital insurance coverage, and government insurance programs were not designed to finance comprehensive care provided on an out of hospital basis.

In order to think sensibly and specifically about how these unacceptable costs can be contained, it is worth considering briefly what these costs represent and how they rose so unexpectedly. As I have already indicated, the increasing sophistication of medicine, its technologies, and its hospitals led to modern care becoming progressively more expensive. As these costs exceeded the range that most people could handle, insurance mechanisms were developed both to protect individuals and to provide the stable financial base necessary to continue to improve our hospitals and advance medical technology.[6] The private health insurance sector grew, and two new medically oriented government insurance programs were established during the 1960s as part of the legislation of the Great Society—one to offset medical care expenses for the aged (Medicare) and the other to provide medical assistance to the poor (Medicaid). Expanded private and public insurance markedly increased the number of dollars flowing to the health sector. However, few foresaw a decade ago that simply changing the way Americans paid for their care would result in such a phenomenal takeoff in the costs of health care. It was generally believed at that time that doctors, hospitals, and nursing homes would merely be paid from a different pocket. However, once the financial barriers to obtaining care had been partially removed by such insurance, health institutions began to behave quite differently. As new funds were made available, a rapid inflationary spiral began. Hospitals take the lion's share of the health care dollar. As monies became available, hospitals began to build, adding beds at a rapid rate to accommodate what they expected would be a greatly increased demand. Second, in response to an anticipated shortage of health professionals, they made available more training opportunities for physicians and nurses and began to pay them adequate salaries. They also rapidly increased both the numbers and the wages of hospital workers, who had traditionally been grossly underpaid. Third, they provided much more care for the poor and the elderly, in response to the national commitment to make health care a right for all citizens regardless of income. Fourth, they moved rapidly to increase their expensive medical technology to provide more accurate diagnosis and treatment, thereby strengthening their abilities to take sophisticated care of hospitalized people.

The costs for these changes—increasing the size of facilities, delivering more services to more people, increasing modern technology, hiring more people to deliver services, and paying adequate wages—all coupled with overall inflation, represent most of the increased costs in the health sector. How these costs can be contained without erasing the advances made represents a serious national problem. There seems little inclination to dismantle our high technology units, to downgrade the training of health professionals, or to return to more primitive forms of care. It seems equally unlikely that hospitals will refuse to care for the poor or reduce the salaries of hospital workers or young physicians. Clearly we should seek to use our physicians and nurses, our hospitals, and our modern procedures as selectively and as wisely as possible, but there are few who would wish to abandon the advances that have been made in the last decade.

THE REMAINING PROBLEMS OF ACCESS TO CARE

While we have made significant improvements in getting many more Americans the medical services they need and in reducing inequities in care available to different income and racial groups, two problems of access remain. First, some special groups of people—special because of age or income or location or type of infirmity—continue to have problems in obtaining adequate amounts of the kinds of care they need. Second, for some people, the care that we know how to give is either unavailable, inappropriate, or falls short of what we now know how to do because we have not organized it properly. Here I wish to document these problems in more detail for reasons that are relatively straightforward. If we can agree that there are special groups who need care and get a clear picture of the nature of the problem and determine its magnitude, we can attack these problems quite specifically, rather than scattering our efforts on the overall issue of access to care. The problems that remain appear of containable size and something that we can get our hands on. A minority, not a majority, of Americans are having difficulty getting medical care.

Directing our efforts at correcting specific shortfalls would be far less costly and more easily accomplished than making global attacks on less well-defined problems. With the global approach, we run the risk of simply scattering our efforts and our monies all over the map, putting many of our resources where they are not needed, and conceivably ending up with the same groups still lacking access to proper medical care. We also need to look more closely at what is available for those who hurdle the access barrier. Do we have the right kinds of health professionals and institutions out there? Are they appropriately distributed? Are we employing our high cost technologies properly? Can we organize care differently to do the job more effectively at less cost? Are we tackling the emotional problems of illness as well as the physiologic ones? Let us look at each of these problems in more detail.

Access for Whom?

There are five groups of Americans whose medical care deserves concerted efforts to improve it—poor children, the poor elderly, our rural citizens, people with chronic illnesses requiring long-term care, and those with permanent physical and mental handicaps that tend to isolate them from the mainstream of American life.

These groups all have some characteristics in common. For one reason or another, be it their age, their helplessness, their dependency, or their isolation, they need help from others to get them to needed services or to get the needed services to them. Our medical care system, structured as it is to deal primarily with acute life crises, is not well designed for such problems. Once proper care or management has been planned, they need other people to help them carry out the plan; they cannot do it alone. Much of the task here is organizational. We need different kinds of programs or special new systems involving the use of other kinds of people to help these groups.

To me, our failure to bring needed medical care to these particular groups of Americans says something sad about the erosion of human support systems in the United States. As families have fragmented, as church life has become less important, and as other human support groups have dwindled or disassembled, these people have tended to be forgotten or ignored. They need other "helpers" to get the care and support they need, and we are not supplying this kind of people. I think we have the resources and the ingenuity to do it, and at prices the nation can afford. Let us examine the nature of the problems experienced by each of these groups.

The Problems of Poor Children. Neglect of childhood health problems can produce profound and often permanent stunting or warping. Our failure to detect and remedy certain early childhood problems places an enormous financial and social burden on society. The consequences of an untreated remediable health problem can be far-reaching. That an untreated middle ear infection can lead to communication difficulties, school failure, sociopathic behavior, and unsatisfactory adulthood seems well documented. Recently, the superintendent of schools of a medium-sized, largely blue collar town told me a story that brought the magnitude of such neglect home very forcefully. In 1974, his school system gave comprehensive reading examinations to 2,500 graduating high school seniors. The results were discouraging. Ten percent, or fully 250 young men and women, were "functionally illiterate," a most serious handicap in our modern world. Similar results have been recorded in many cities, but this school system went further. They gave medical examinations to 50 percent of those 250 graduates who did so poorly. To their dismay, the majority were shown to have readily detectable medical problems. Poor vision, poor hearing, and mental retardation were common. The most devastating finding was that 90 percent of these "illiterate" children had been in that same school system since grade one. Thus, one of our social institutions had had responsibility for these children for twelve years without recognizing what was wrong. To its credit, this city has now put a whole new system of medical detection and care into operation in its schools to try to prevent this dreadful waste of human potential.[7]

Two-thirds of all children now live in metropolitan areas. Approximately one out of four, or seventeen million youngsters, live in poverty, and almost one of every two black children is poor. This is coupled with a lack of support for parents in their child-rearing role caused by the increasing fragmentation of families and the relative isolation of many parents from other social groups. Today one-half of all mothers with school age children hold jobs outside the home. One out of six children now lives in a single parent family, and in certain inner city areas, Harlem, for instance, almost one out of two children has only one parent at home and frequently no one during working hours.[8]

Some of the studies on poor inner city children reveal a shocking neglect of remediable problems. An Institute of Medicine study of poor Washington children showed that 25 percent of those between the ages of six months and two years had anemia. More than 25 percent about to go to school failed comprehensive vision exams. About 20 percent had overt middle ear disease, and 7 percent had hearing losses in the speech frequency range serious enough to interfere with learning. More than 50 percent of the black children in the survey had not even been immunized against poliomyelitis.[9] Bear in mind that these are all medical problems that we know well how to treat. In a wealthy nation that purports to care a great deal about giving all its children a fair run at life, these statistics seem inexcusable.

To these problems must be added a whole new set of childhood problems currently coming into medical purview. These have either been unmasked as many of the infectious disease killer of children have disappeared from the scene or have emerged as the unwanted accompaniment of our changing society. Today a disturbing number of school age children—estimates run as high as 30 percent—are described as having "learning" or "behavioral" difficulties.[10] These children are hyperactive or belligerent, destructive to themselves or to others. These behavioral aberrations were not previously considered medical problems, but there is increasing evidence to suggest that some stem from underlying neurologic or physiologic dysfunction undetected early in life. All evidence points to such dysfunctions as important predictors of subsequent life failure, and society pays an enormous price for ignoring them. Certain studies suggest that they can be spotted very early, perhaps by age four. There is tentative evidence that certain kinds of interventions, certain ways of treating these problems early, can make a difference. Clearly we would be foolish and shortsighted if we did not move aggressively to try to tailor our medical care system to do just this.

Despite the overall improvement in access to physician care that have been made during the last decade, low income children have made disappointing gains. While the gap has narrowed, in 1976 poor children saw physicians 23 percent less often than children from middle or high income families. To date, we have not succeeded in moving poor children into the mainstream of American medical care. We need to do so.

The Problems of the Elderly Poor. It is well known that we are witnessing a steady, indeed accelerating, shift toward a society composed of more older people. In the United States in 1975 slightly over 10 percent of the population, 22.3 million people, were above the age of sixty-five. This group is projected to increase to almost thirty million before the year 2000. Within this group, as might be anticipated, there are a large number who are poor, and the incidence of disease or illness that significantly impairs performance is appreciable.[11] Over 11 percent of those between the ages of sixty-five and seventy-five cannot function independently because of physical or emotional infirmities. The incidence of this dependency, generally due to illness, rises sharply to almost 60 percent for those who are seventy-five or older. At all ages, the rates of disability for those who are poor are almost double those of people from higher income groups. Here again, those who are poor are lagging behind, despite their greater need for proper medical care to maintain independent function. Although the descrepancies in physician visits between those elderly who are poor and those who are not is less dramatic than is the case with children, they exist and have grown worse during the last decade. In 1976 the poor elderly, with twice as much disability as their financially better off contemporaries, saw physicians 7.5 percent less frequently.

We are currently spending very large sums of money for the care of the frail or infirm elderly. Almost 36 percent of our national health expenditures are directed at this 10 percent of the population. However, the ways in which we make these expenditures and the quality of the care received leave much to be desired. Most of this care is institutional and is either crisis-oriented or custodial. A worrisome number of our acute medical and surgical hospital beds are occupied by older people, many with problems that might have been avoided by better organized and oriented out of hospital services. Over one million—or 5 percent of the elderly—reside in institutions, mostly proprietary nursing homes, which, as a group, are among the most depressing and dehumanizing places to house ("warehouse" would be a more appropriate word in some cases) human beings who are unable to fend for themselves. In a number of states, the Medicaid budget—the funds made available by the public sector to pay for the care of the poor of all ages—represents the single largest budgetary item, and some of these states are spending over 50 percent of this budget on nursing home costs. Clearly there are better ways of dealing with the problems of the illness and infirmities of the aged, and we should get at them, if for none other than the self-interested reason that eventually being old will be the eventual lot of all of us.

Problems of Rural Dwellers. Rural dwellers continue to have major problems in obtaining their share of prompt and appropriate medical services. The discrepancy in visits made to physicians between those in urban and those in rural areas has actually widened during the past decade. Part of this is due to the progressive urbanization of our population and a corresponding decline in the number of physicians who have chosen to practice in rural areas. Part of the gap is due to a disparity in health care financing between urban and rural areas. Both public and private health insurance programs continue to make it financially more attractive for health professionals to practice in urban communities.[12]

Problems of the Chronically Ill. This fourth group is separated from others not by age or income but by the misfortune of having chronic, long-term disabling illness. Medicine as it is now practiced is at its best in the management of acute or life-threatening illness. Here events take place in rapid sequence. Initial physician involvement is intense, and his actions are frequently definitive. Giving antibiotics and oxygen to the patient with pneumonia, administering blood transfusions and sedation to the patient with massive bleeding, or setting a broken bone are examples of such actions. In our modern world, however, these problems occupy only a small amount of most physicians' time. Instead, a number of more chronic long-term problems contribute very significantly to the load on the medical care system. Here the physician's efforts cannot be definitive, and what the physician does represents only a small fraction of the total effort required to obtain a satisfactory outcome. Thus, in diseases like hypertension, chronic lung disease, diabetes, or crippling arthritis, the medical services currently delivered are often found wanting.

These diseases have some features in common that make their management difficult for both parties involved—patients and health professionals alike. First, the disease or condition is often asymptomatic for long periods before producing overt illness or disability.

However, these diseases are often forerunner of serious illness. Some, notably hypertension, obesity, and perhaps certain form of chronic lung disease, are susceptible to preventive interventions if they are detected early and if proper measures are applied. Second, once they have developed, these diseases and conditions are lifetime affairs. While treatment and plans for disease management are available to prevent or ameliorate the illness these diseases can produce, once started, therapy must be continued for long periods, often for life. To stay on such regimens is difficult. The medicines may be unpleasant or the restrictions imposed difficult to live with. To stick with such a program of therapy, the patient needs much encouragement; the long-term benefits of staying with the treatment need continuous reinforcement. Minor variations in management can be all-important. But the physician is simply not close at hand each day, every month, every year, to make these adjustments or to stiffen the patient's resolve. Although the physician can diagnose these chronic problems and can generally indicate what should be done, he is simply not in a position to do much more than that. As a consequence, the benefits of medical knowledge are not really brought to bear on the patient's condition. For management to be successful, very different strategies and very different organizational arrangements are required than those that are suitable for acute or self-limiting illnesses. To date we have not adequately addressed the failures of the medical system in coping with these burdensome illnesses that are so prevalent today. It is clear that medicine alone and physicians working in one-on-one relationships with patients cannot deal with these conditions. Solutions to this problem are not mysterious or expensive: we need new alliances and new strategies to better apply what we know.

Problems of the Handicapped. Last on my list of individuals who as a group have special problems in access to care are those with handicaps of sufficient severity to make their entry into the medical care system—indeed, into most aspects of American life—awkward, difficult, or impossible without assistance from others. There are conservatively 2.5 million Americans of working age with disabilities so severe that they are totally unable to earn an income as society is now structured. Roughly 7.6 million are classified as disabled by virtue of confinement to wheelchair, blindness, cerebral palsy, or other forms of severe handicap.[13] Clearly, medical care is but one of multiple problems these individuals find in gaining access to American life. We have forgotten them in the design of our public buildings, elevators, toilet facilities, and public transportation. The same applies to our hospitals and to physicians' and dentists' offices. The Rehabilitation Act of 1973 recognizes this oversight and mandates that all institutions and programs receiving federal assistance bring these individuals into employment or programs or services where barriers now exist to their entry. We need to examine our medical care services to be sure that they are accessible to the handicapped.

This, then, is the first half of the access problem. These are the groups that require our special attention. The other half of the access problem is access to what. Here again, the problems seem approachable.

Access to What?

Although we are beginning to address this problem, we continue to have a serious misfit between the kinds of physicians most agree should be available to handle the common medical problems in American society and the kinds of physicians that are actually trained and available. For the reasons outlined in Chapter 2, until very recently there has been a steady decline in the number of physicians electing to enter general practice and an increasing number trained as specialists. Obviously, many of the general medical care needs of Americans have been assumed by physicians with specialist labels, primarily internists, pediatricians, and to a lesser extent, obstetricians-gynecologists and even psychiatrists. This has proved unsatisfactory, in part because it is largely a hidden system and makes projections and planning for national health manpower frustrating and difficult. A worrisome geographic maldistribution of physicians and other health professionals also contributes to problems of access. We are not alone in this difficulty; geographic inequities in the availability of health professionals is a problem that troubles virtually every other country in the Western world. The magnitude of the discrepancy in the numbers of health professionals in rural areas, particularly in the South or in inner city ghetto areas, vis-à-vis the more affluent suburbs of major cities has caused serious resentment and much criticism. While the Boston area can claim 239 physicians per 100,000 residents, certain rural areas have fewer than 45 doctors per 100,000 people. The state of New York has 228 physicians per 100,000 residents; the state of Mississippi has only 82.[14] Similar differences between the numbers of physicians in suburbia and in the inner city can be cited for many of our metropolises. These kinds of data on kinds, numbers, and distribution of physicians and other health professionals do not really tell us what we wish to know—the adequacy of care received by people residing in particular areas. The ratio of physicians to population has no necessary relationship either to the quality of services or to health. Thus, those who argue for the status quo are fond of pointing out that health indices for New York and Nebraska are similar, despite an enormous disparity in the number of physicians per population in the two states. The physician to population ratio is, however, one yardstick for assessing the potential availability of medical services, and certainly a 500 percent variation in physician density suggests that we are not optimumly distributing our health professionals.

There is also much to indicate that the quality of patient-health professional interaction needs more of our attention. Medical care varies widely in promptness, appropriateness, dignity, and compassion. The majority of the well to do receive their medical care in private settings—in the physician's office, in the home, or in telephone conversations with their doctor. The poor receive a much greater proportion of their care from other sources—from hospital outpatient departments, from health clinics, and more recently from what have been branded "Medicaid mills." The quality and content of these interactions need more attention if one physician visit is actually to equal another.

While I have in the main emphasized that one of our major lacks is generalist care, we also need much better ways for ensuring that people with special kinds of problems requiring special kinds of services will get the care they need. The pregnant woman at high risk needs not generalist care, but entry into a sophisticated system of perinatal care that will supply her with the care that our medical technology can now give to guarantee a healthy infant and mother. Patients with certain forms of cancer such as leukemia or Hodgkins disease need prompt transfer to highly sophisticated technologic centers where their needs can be much better served.

We also need to organize our system of medical care to make more conservative and more appropriate use of the technologies available. There is much to suggest that the availability of highly sophisticated technologies prompts us to overuse them.[15] There is also reason to believe that we sometimes divert medical resources to very costly care like cardiac bypass surgery without being sure that it pays off, while ignoring the proven and cost-effective use of our finite resources for such preventive interventions as immunizations and prenatal care. In addition, many of our old and some of our new technologies have been introduced quite widely in medical practice before they have been properly validated. They have greatly increased the cost of medical care, frequently caused patient discomfort, and sometimes themselves produced illness. We often proceed to employ them with insufficient evidence that they improve medical care or health. There seems little question that we use our costly technologic tools extravagantly, that we overprescribe drugs, that we may do fair amounts of surgery that may not be necessary, and that we are currently practicing medicine in ways that are needlessly expensive. We hospitalize patients for diagnostic studies that could be done on an ambulatory basis, and we do too many of them. We buy too many CAT scanners, cobalt units, linear accelerators, and other costly devices that could be regionally allocated, and we underutilize them. We have too many underused obstetrical units and empty pediatric beds in many areas. We need to match better actual medical needs with medical resources if we are to make our medical care system more efficient.

This, then, is my list of remaining problems that need our focused attention. It is not really a particularly long list. In the next chapter I will offer some recommendations about how we might begin to address these problems.

Chapter 4

Tackling the Unfinished Agenda

If the remaining unsolved problems in delivering medical care to all Americans are indeed as circumscribed as I have indicated, is their solution a simple matter? Obviously the answer is no. If this were the case, we would have eliminated the shortfalls long ago. Keeping the costs of medical care within acceptable limits and finding ways of delivering better care to those particular groups now lagging behind the rest of us have been the focus of the labors of many dedicated people for many years, yet the problems remain with us. Six years of working on these issues have made me vividly aware of the enormously complex circumstances that often block progress in dealing with these deceptively simple problems.

But we can make a start. Rather than offering global solutions, let me simply list some first steps that might begin to move us in appropriate directions.

RESTRAINING THE ESCALATION OF THE COSTS OF MEDICAL CARE

I am not an economist; thus, here I tread on shaky ground. However, I have not seen any master plan or examples of health care systems in other nations that have magically made medical care inexpensive. Modern medical care will continue to cost a lot, and my readings of American priorities suggest that we are willing to place a significant number of our dollars in this area. What costs money and why has been quite clearly identified, and I believe we will opt to continue our sophisticated system of medicine. Clearly we are not going to dismantle our hospitals, although we could find ways of eliminating beds that are no longer needed. We are not going to abandon our modern medical technology, though we may be able to learn how to use it more selectively and with more restraint. We are not going to pay lower wages to workers in the health industry, though we may find ways of deploying the time and talents of our expensive health professionals more wisely and efficiently. There·are, however, three important steps that could be taken to slow the escalation of costs so that they are more in line with our general economy.

1. We should put major emphasis on improving ways to deliver care on an ambulatory basis and reduce inpatient hospital care.
2. We should increase our efforts to train more physicians for generalist careers, make such careers professionally and financially more attractive, and train new physicians to recognize better the financial implications of the care they render.
3. We should accelerate our efforts to regionalize high technology, underutilized services, and services for certain special groups with special problems, while forging regional linkages to cover better those areas now sparsely supplied with health professionals.

Let me explain each of these three proposals in somewhat greater detail.

Strengthening Ambulatory Care.   Our use of hospitals and the increasing cost of the care provided therein is the single factor that contributes the most to our escalating expenses. Our hospitalization rates are nearly the highest in the world, and it is in hospitals that very expensive technologies are most often used. If we could shift the incentives so that physicians and patients alike found it to their advantage to manage illnesses out of hospital, a significant brake might be put on rising medical care costs. (As a simple example, merely cutting one day from the hospital stay of all patients admitted last year would have saved this nation approximately $2 billion.) To do this will require that we design our insurance programs to cover the costs of ambulatory care. Without such coverage, all other efforts to move care out of the hospital will fail.

At the same time, it makes sense to encourage the establishment of arrangements in which physicians assume responsibility for the total and continuing care of defined population groups. Both prepaid plans and plans that combine prepayment and fee for service seem to have this potential. The evidence is abundant that plans in which physicians and/or institutions make such a commitment to the continuous care of a group of people are highly effective in reducing hospitalization rates. Indeed, such evidence prompted the health maintenance organization (HMO) legislation. Nationally, there are an average of five hospitals beds per 1,000 people. Kaiser Permanente—a prepaid plan—maintains two beds per 1,000 enrollees. Rate of hospitalization in this particular program average only 30 to 60 percent of that of the population at large. The reduction in beds maintained for Kaiser Permanente subscribers profoundly reduces the numbers and the costs of hospital employees as well. For every bed not maintained, we eliminate the need for five hospital employees per 1,000 people. Organization of fee for service physicians in new ways to deliver services to particular groups may be able to similiarly reduce costs.[1] Hospitals that need to fill their beds to stay solvent and employees who need the jobs will not view this recommendation with enthusiasm. However, giving more care in ambulatory settings seems the only practical long-range solution to our national problem of too rapidly escalating health care costs.

Training More Generalist Physicians and Making New Doctors Better Aware of the Cost Implications of Their Diagnostic and Therapeutic Acts. If we are to move responsibly to giving more medical care outside of the hospital, we need to be certain that we have enough skilled physicians who can operate effectively and comfortably in this setting. We have too few of them today. As I will indicate in Chapter 6, academic medical center faculties, composed largely of specialists with little contact with primary care problems or out of hospital patients, currently do a poor job of preparing aspiring physicians for a generalist role. Major efforts to correct this are now afoot. Programs to train family practitioners have been growing rapidly, fueled by federal mandate and funds. Whereas there were only 146 programs to train family physicians and general practitioners in 1966, there were 346 by 1976. At the same time, a number of academic centers are recasting their residency training programs to develop genuine primary care tracks for those who will become internists and pediatricians. To date, the movement in these directions has been slow, however. Current training programs in primary care are regarded as not as rigorous or sophisticated as they might be, and the full creativity of the academic world has simply not been brought to bear on how to make generalist careers as professionally challenging and rewarding as those of specialists.

To accomplish this more swiftly, academic medical centers need to develop more realistic settings in which such education can be carried out. (See Chapter 7 for a fuller discussion of this proposal.)

Academic centers must bite off a real piece of the ambulatory care action and commit themselves to manageable responsibilities for the total care of defined groups of people. This entails a quite different approach from simply holding office hours in outpatient departments. It means that academic institutions would have to accept full responsibility for delivering comprehensive care to a particular group of people twenty-four hours a day, 365 days a year. It is my conviction that if an academic medical institution and its faculty, house staff, and students have genuine nondelegatable responsibilities for this very real kind of general care, they will move briskly and imaginatively to make generalist careers all that they should be. I believe they will find ways of enriching and refining the content of general practice in so doing and will thus make such careers more attractive to new graduates.

Increasing the number of generalist physicians will also require changing the financial incentives that help dictate career choices in medicine. The dedicated general internist or family practitioner working in a rural area now receives significantly less remuneration than the specialist who practices fewer hours in a major hospital. If we really wish to move more effective medical care out into the community, we will have to correct this financial imbalance.

I believe it is also necessary to give physicians a better understanding of the financial implications of the medical care they prescribe and deliver. In the final analysis, it will be enormously difficult to contain expenditures for medical care without changing the behavior of the individual who creates most of the costs—the physician. Almost 80 percent of in-hospital costs are generated by physicians' decision about the use of facilities, drugs, or technologies. A number of studies have shown that each new doctor who is added to the pool of practicing physicians generates between $200,000 and $350,000 in health care expenses each year. A family physician who recently kept careful track of the health care costs he himself created by his decisions and actions found that these amounted to $13,400 in the course of a single day![3]

To suggest that the physician be trained to consider the financial implications of each of his acts and to consider alternative ways of approaching problems may be more practical than it seems at first. The larger output of our medical schools today means that over 60,000 new physicians will enter the workforce during the next four years. This will represent almost one-quarter of the total physicians in practice. Consequently any change in the outlook approach of the young men and women who are now becoming doctors should over a reasonable time period have a significant impact. My tougher-minded economist colleagues feel that the system must also contain real incentives for physicians to cut these costs. This can be done when groups of physicians contract for the care of groups of patients for a predetermined amount of money, but making physicians better aware of the costs and benefits of alternative courses of action is a step. Anyway, it is worth a try, and some institutions are now experimenting with it.

Regionalizing High Technology, Low Usage Services, Regionalizing Special Programs for Special Groups; Developing Regional Linkages to Offset Geographic Maldistribution of Health Professionals. Some of our remarkable new technologies should serve as potent incentives for regionalization. The duplication of certain kinds of high cost, low usage services in each and every hospital simply cannot be justified or continued. We must, as a nation, decide how many CAT scanners, cobalt treatment units, open heart surgery units, and the like are required to fulfill patient needs in particular regions of the country. We must then make some tough decisions about who shall and who shall not have these pieces of equipment and services. These decisions will require great wisdom and tact. They should be made, if possible, in ways that will not blight individual institutional pride or initiative. We must at the same time develop more effective methods for validating the effectiveness of high cost technologies before they are broadly introduced upon the national scene. In the process, we should reassess the effectiveness of some of the expensive technologies already in place. Are intensive care units really effective in reducing mortality? Does coronary bypass surgery contribute to the quality of life—does it extend it—for those who have had heart attacks? Decisions regarding technology—both its usefulness and its deployment—will not be easy. Without such decisions, however, we will either block the progress of medicine, condemning it to continue many practices now agreed to be inadequate, or continue the rapid escalation of its costliness.

Strategies for the regional organization of services could have other advantages in addition to restraining costs. First, regionalization would help address the problem of the geographic maldistribution of health professionals, which will probably always be with us. Second, it seems a way of developing better systems of care for special groups and special problems that require mobilization of resources above and beyond what an individual practitioner can offer. Academic medical centers have already been much involved in attempting to offer on a regional basis the special services that they are uniquely able to deliver. I believe that we must also much better utilize our network of almost 7,000 community hospitals to better answer the health care needs of regions. Better linkages between these institutions and colleagues in the field seem a logical next step. In inner cities, where municipal and metropolitan hospitals are sometimes virtually the only major institutions left standing, linking satellite ambulatory units to these hospitals seems the only sensible route to go. In rural areas, linkages to hospitals are critically important if rural practitioners are to maintain their skills and to find professional life in isolated communities viable and rewarding.

It has also long seemed to me that various powerful professional groups—the specialty academies and specialist and generalist societies—could also participate more vigorously in solving problems of access. Why couldn't all the pediatricians in a given region collectively agree to organize and operate a program that would guarantee all children in their region, regardless of race, income, or location, full immunization—or that all vision and hearing and other remedial problems would be detected and managed? Similarly, I see no reason why the obstetrician-gynecologists of a given area could not reach similar agreements about their responsibilities for the prenatal, delivery, and postnatal care of all pregnant women in their region, regardless of a patient's location or ability to pay. Such voluntary actions of responsible professional groups would seem vastly preferable to yet more centralization of such responsibilities. Medical care is a very personalized form of service, and solution to the problems of distributing care equally and meeting the requirements of special groups will be much more satisfactory and permanent if they are planned and designed for the unique needs of a particular region and are voluntarily carried out.

I make these suggestions because I am persuaded that the geographic maldistribution of health professionals will never be completely overcome. It is worth pointing out that countries that have nationalized payment mechanisms or even nationalized health services have not resolved this problem satisfactorily, although a number have done better than we do. As transportation improves and as we move toward more sophisticated regionalization of services, geographic distances from health professionals and facilities may not represent as significant a barrier to obtaining care as they have in the past and currently do, but the special problems of underserved areas will always require careful planning and attention. One way of solving the problem of underdoctored areas that is now gaining momentum is to agree that serving as a physician in a generalist capacity in an underserved area for a specified period is simply part of the contract each young man or woman who elects to become a doctor makes upon entering medical school. The National Health Service Corps is one such program, though perhaps it does not go far enough. A two year commitment of each graduate to work in an area designated as underserved would not seem to me an unacceptable burden to place on those fortunate enough to enter medicine. Such an experience might even cause some to opt to continue their practice in such settings. These young doctors could enter such service after one year of postgraduate training and be salaried by the government. Such national service might be a prerequisite for entry into any specialty training program. It would not fully answer the needs of communities for continuing care, but it is worth pointing out that many physicians had a similar obligation in the armed services in years past, and that wartime medical care was handled with considerable effectiveness, despite the fact that physicians served limited time periods.

There will continue to be some communities too small, too remote, or too sparsely populated to sustain a physician. Here the nurse practitioner, physician assistant, or other health professional, working under physician supervision from afar, seem the only logical answer. Improved communications technology and transportation should make linkages to physicians and backup resources progressively easier. Audiovisual linkages between hospitals and the remote locales served by these new health professionals are well within our reach; they are already in use in certain areas. How these individuals function in practice settings has been more carefully studied and documented than have any of the services performed by physicians. That they can do the job and do it well seems solidly established.

Improving Access To and the Kinds of Care Received by Groups Out of the Mainstream of American Medicine

Some of the approaches suggested for curbing runaway medical care expenses—focusing on out of hospital care, putting more generalists in place, and regionalizing expensive or special services—should in the process improve the distribution and equity of medical services deployed. But the special needs of the special groups now inadequately served that I have described will require more precisely directed efforts. The fact that we have already made such remarkable strides in improving access to medical care for many who were previously underserved shows that we can accomplish more if we plan for it and work toward it. The reasons for improving medical care for these special groups seem to me logical and straightforward. First, and most basically, it simply seems right. We have had a long tradition in this country of helping those who are unable to help themselves. It is in keeping with our American ethic to do so here.

Second, as I view it, this is a manageable task. Developing programs that will bring these special groups of Americans into the medical care system is well within what we can afford. Access to medical care is no longer a problem for the majority of Americans—only a relatively small number still need attention. Last of all, I am concerned that should we fail to recognize that it is simply these particular groups with their particular problems that remain outside the system, we may continue to put enormous amounts of money into addressing a broader problem that is no longer there. We may scatter our resources too widely, only to find that we have not reached those who most need our help.

What then is needed? The answers are deceptively simple. We need to get these special groups to the care they require or get the care to them. In order to do this we must organize medical care differently, to suit the special needs of these particular groups.

The central problem that blocks the entry of all of the groups I have discussed into the medical care system is their inability to find their way into it by themselves. This problem has been caused in part by the progressive fragmentation of American family life, the dissolution of the extended family, and the atrophy of other social institutions that formerly shared responsibility for those less fortunate. Medicine has the know-how to give all of these groups a richer and more fulfilling life. We simply need to find foolproof ways of seeing that they get it. They need families or advocates or helpers or life-supporters; they need either transportation to services or services brought to them. These are jobs that need not be done by health professionals, or even by paid employees. Here I believe we must plan better ways of systematically harnessing man's basic tendency to help others. In a recent editorial, Gorernor Brown of California pointed out that if we actually took all of the jobs that need doing in service fields and put salaried people to work on them, we would generate astronomical costs and still have nowhere near enough people to fill those jobs.[4] We need to reestablish or, better harness the voluntarism that has traditionally characterized our American society and to organize it in sensible ways to help bring care to our children, our elderly, our handicapped, and our chronically ill. We need individuals or groups who can pinch-hit when families are unable to be responsible for their children or their elderly or the handicapped. In a society that worries about the lack of meaningful roles for teenagers or the relative isolation of the retired elderly, why not make use of these groups? With simple training and minimal funding, many teenagers, widows or widowers, and healthy but lonely elderly could be enlisted to bring such people into the system.

They could serve as physician extenders, reinforcing and modulating the care needed and establishing a life support system of mutual benefit to both the server and the served. Developing such service roles for those now lacking meaningful tasks in our world would have a warm and human quality that could soften some of the harshness of modern life and might permit new mutually supportive groupings. These are not complicated or mysterious roles—but they might be of enormous importance to us in improving the quality of modern society.

Although there are certain problems shared in common by all of the special groups now lacking such care, there are specific strategies that could improve care for each particular groups.

Improving the Care of Poor Children. First, we need better financing of health care for children. Dr. Theodore Marmor, a political scientist, has suggested that the obvious place to begin in any national health insurance scheme is the development of full financing for the care of children and expectant women.[5] I concur. Clearly, financial want should be no barrier to the most effective preventive and remedial care we can offer children. Furthermore, comprehensive medical care for children costs relatively little. They are a basically healthy population, and the payoffs from prevention and remedial intervention are considerable.

We have a number of institutions already in place to which we might logically tie child health programs. The school system is the most obvious one. Several imaginative programs have shown that using schools as a base for specially trained nurses and funding such programs with public monies that are already available can result in a comprehensive and highly effective medical care program for youngsters, irrespective of income. To make such programs fully effective, however, we would have to change our customs regarding when the school and the child initiate their relationship. Many studies suggest that the detection or the correction of childhood defects by the time of school entry is much too late. We need to direct more aggressive attention to the health needs of children during the first few years of life. Hence there are some interesting straws in the wind. One cooperative program initiated by The Children's Hospital Medical Center and the city of Brookline, Massachusetts, now registers children with the school and a health system upon birth. The children and their families are regularly examined and given appropriate medical and educational assistance from birth until entry into the school system. While this experimental program is presently very expensive, it is demonstrating some interesting and exciting possibilities for giving children the best start that modern society can offer.[6]

Daycare centers—another spot where youngsters from poor backgrounds are often congregated—seem like another logical place to deliver diagnostic and treatment services for preschool children. Other youth organizations could also be possible sites for the delivery of both health and medical services. YMCAs and YWCAs, the Boy Scouts and Girl Scouts, 4-H Clubs, and so forth seem logical organizations to assist families in getting their children the medical care and health information they require. In many child care programs, the use of health professionals other than the physician—the nurse-practitioner, the health advocate, the home visitor—has been shown to be effective. Most children are basically healthy most of the time. The kinds of immunizations they need are straightforward and well established. Tests for the detection of many defects or potential medical problems can be readily performed by nonphysicians. What are needed are foolproof linkages of such detection systems to physicians and other appropriate medical backup so that the problems uncovered get properly managed. I do not think this too complicated a task for American society to undertake.

Improving Medical Care for the Elderly Poor. Getting the increasing numbers of the aged or infirm who are poor to the medical care they need and deserve poses a tougher problem. There are few places where they come together. They have many more medical problems than children, often chronic, disabling, and expensive. Their care is already consuming large numbers of health care dollars. Our society has not developed satisfactory ways of keeping them productively involved in our world. As with children, they need helpers and advocates, not simply more medical care. They need continuing assistance to carry out plans for the management of their infirmities. We need more ways of maintaining them in the community rather than institutionalizing them.

Here is where I believe developing helping roles for unemployed teenagers, lonely elderly, and others now adrift or invisible in our society deserves real study. Modest sums to train and employ such individuals to help frail elderly remain within the community while receiving the medical attention they need should be cost-effective. Organizing around manageable-sized people units—a city block, a housing development, a village—would seem the way to go. There are experiments already in place in certain communities to build on.

Our nursing homes are, with certain exceptions, a national disgrace. The elderly poor have been ignored or forgotten by most of our society and the medical profession alike. One solution that I have long advocated to bring nursing homes into the mainstream of medical care and thus upgrade their quality is the simple device of mandating that all nursing homes be closely tied to and the responsibility of voluntary hospitals and the physicians who staff those hospitals; each hospital might be obligated to assume responsibilities for its share of nursing home beds. By and large, these institutions are presently outside the medical care system. They might play a very different role if we brought them into it.

Providing Effective Care for the Chronically Ill. The care of long-term, potentially disabling chronic illness that does not kill is a problem with subtly different dimensions. Here we know what to do, but have not designed our system to deal effectively and on a continuing basis with these disease problems. The solutions—or partial solutions—look relatively straightforward. There are relatively few mysteries in the diagnosis of the chronic illnesses that now form a large portion of most medical practices. Congestive heart failure, arthritis, asthma, emphysema, and obesity are generally quickly recognized by both the patient and physician. Hypertension can be diagnosed by anyone with access to a blood pressure cuff, and diabetes by a few simple laboratory procedures.

We cannot at present cure these diseases. We can, however, do much more to permit people to function more effectively despite them. When patients follow the proper regimens, some of the most devastating and crippling aftermaths of these diseases can be prevented. Herein lies the problem. With most of these chronic problems, we are getting only about 20 percent good results because of inadequate application of what we know, whereas medical knowledge should permit us to treat these patients with at least 80 percent effectiveness. Chronic disease problems require well-informed patients, regimens that are rather precisely tailored to patients' particular needs, and the motivation to stick with these regimens. What most patients need is some continuing contact with another interested party to keep what medicine knows how to do properly applied. This party need not be a doctor, but it should be someone who is reasonably knowledgeable about the disease and well acquainted with the person and the treatment. It has been well documented that nurse practitioners can play this role with great success, but it seems probable that in many instances a lesser-trained person can do the job. This health helper can often make modulating course corrections in management and offer the encouragement that frequently can make the difference between a patient's being able to function satisfactorily in society or being condemned to bedridden isolation.

This is a role that the physician simply cannot play, even if constitutionally and emotionally equipped to do so. It takes too much of his or her high-priced time. To manage these kinds of problems, we must design systems that permit medically assisted self-care. In the final analysis, in these kinds of chronic illnesses, the affected individual is the main provider of care. The patient needs the physician to design the regimen, to make necessary modifications when appropriate, and to then place him in a setting that can assist him in becoming a knowledgeable provider-consumer of that care.

To move in this direction would not be new for medicine. Indeed, the effective management of many acute problems in medicine has evolved in just this fashion. In modern acute care, we make use of many people other than physicians in the management of patients. I have recently been living closely with the agonies faced by a young woman severely burned in a flash grease fire. Her initial management—relief of pain, management of shock, replacement of fluids, prevention of infection—was the task of a skillful physician, requiring many of his hours during the first week. However, the problem of her rehabilitation—preventing crippling contractures, administering daily care to the burn sites, exercising her atrophied muscles, helping her relearn how to walk, giving her reassurance and encouragement, and countering the depression caused by months of slow recovery—has been the role of a skilled and supportive physiotherapist. Without the physician, this burn victim might not have survived. Without the physiotherapist, she might have survived as a physical and emotional cripple. She has depended heavily on each of them, and this triangular arrangement of physician-patient-physiotherapist has been critical to her genuine recovery. The analogies here for the better care of those with chronic illness, or the maintenance of the elderly, or the care of children with certain kinds of problems are obvious.

There are now a number of interesting experiments underway that suggest that we can multiply the effective application of medical knowledge by forming better organized alliances between patients, physicians, and other socially responsible people. This has been done with considerable success in the management of hypertension, diabetes, chronic lung disease, and obesity.[7] Such arrangements have permitted physicians and patients to get better mileage from what we know. To date, most of these programs have been categorically oriented. That is, the service is offered only for those with hypertension or multiple sclerosis or another specific disease problem.

Recently, however, my colleague Dr. Leighton Cluff and his associates at The Robert Wood Johnson Foundation have made a careful survey of the kinds of services required by people suffering from a wide variety of chronic disease problems. This survey showed that the services required fell into but a few large groupings. Help with adjustments in medications (diabetes, hypertension, etc.), physiotherapy (arthritis, many neurologic diseases, chronic lung disease), mutual aid groups, home care services, and nursing services led the list. Development of regionally organized units that could offer both physicians and patients such an array of services—units in which our categorically oriented voluntary organizations could also get more for their money—would seem a logical next step. Such programs could add much to the effectiveness of medical care and the quality of life for many Americans with chronic problems and could do it at costs that were acceptable to society.

Providing Better Medical Care for the Handicapped. Much of what I have suggested in the foregoing sections could also be applied to the delivery of better medical care to the handicapped—another group too often ignored in current society. But here the problem has yet another facet to it. Because many physicians and most dentists lack experience with the handicapped during medical and dental training, they are uncomfortable with—indeed, somewhat afraid of—taking on these people as patients. For example, most of the patients with severe neurologic or musculoskeletal handicaps that I have cared for have had dreadful untended dental problems, simply because dentists have been unwilling to see them in their offices. Early experience with the handicapped, allowing those who give care to feel more comfortable with them, needs more attention by the institutions that educate health professionals. It is now being addressed by some dental schools, but medicine and nursing must start to look at this problem more carefully as well.

Improving the "Texture" of the Doctor-Patient Interaction. Last, I believe those in medicine must better use the potent therapeutic potential of the physician "caring" for the patient in strengthening what medicine can offer to our society. Emotional access as well as physical access to care is important to people who consult doctors. Over the past ten to fifteen years, however, I have perceived a gradual erosion in this facet of the physician-patient relationship. In part this seems to stem from society's demystification of the doctor; in part it stems from our technologic successes.

It almost seems that as we have developed ways of doing more to patients that beneficially affects outcome, we tend to care for him or her less. The quality of the interaction between a sick person and a potential healer needs more attention by medicine today.

The feeling of distance between one person and another is hardly unique to medicine. One sees it in interactions between store clerks and customers, bus drivers and bus riders, taxi drivers and their fares, teachers and their students. A lack of willingness to reach out to others or to engage with them in positive ways pervades modern society. Physicians have a potentially powerful role to play in redressing this problem in their interactions with those to whom they give care. They remain strong models for others, and the ways in which they conduct their human relationships often have ripple effects far wider than those resulting from a particular one-on-one transaction. This is an area that can only be addressed by the profession and the institutions that develop physicians. How medicine is offered to those requesting it could be a potent and unifying force in shaping a world that is less angry, less anxious, and more human. I will have more to say on this subject in Part III of this book.

This, then, is where I come out in the year 1978. We have much that is good within our system of medical care on which we can build. We have developed the most sophisticated and technologically advanced methods for managing serious or life-threatening illness to be found anywhere in the world. We have an adequate number of hospitals, they are generally of good quality, and they form a respectable network on which to build new programs. We are training more than enough doctors, nurses, and other health professionals to supply adequate care to all if we deploy them appropriately and if we make better use of other people not ordinarily considered part of the health care system.

During the last decade, we have made real improvements in getting people to physicians, and we have narrowed the gap between the amounts of care received by the well to do and by those who are poor or from minority backgrounds. We have shown that better organization of care for certain special groups—notably children, pregnant women, and people with special disease problems—can reduce costs, morbidity, mortality, and the burden of chronic illness.

Occurring in parallel with the above—but with absolutely no data to suggest that the two are interrelated—we have some gross indicators that the health of Americans is improving. This is manifested by falling age-adjusted death rates, improved infant and maternal mortality statistics, declining death rates from coronary artery disease, indeed, decreased death rates for eleven of the leading fifteen causes of death in the United States. These encouraging changes should give us the confidence necessary to move on with the unfinished agenda. Medical care is expensive and becoming more-so. We must curb the inflationary spiral of costs which threatens to divert us from others of equal human importance, and I have suggested some ways of tackling this problem.

We now need to direct attention to getting certain special groups who have special health and medical problems to the care they need. We know what is required, but we need to organize and deploy both medical personnel and others differently to effect it.

To accomplish these tasks, we need to realize that these steps to improve our society take time and patience and the cooperative efforts of many. We are an impatient people, with much energy but a short attention span. As a nation, we need to recognize how long our present advances have taken, agree that we have within ourselves and our institutions the capacity to improve access to medical care for those citizens who still lack it, and roll up our sleeves and get on with the task.

✳ *Part II*

The Academic Medical Center:
A Stressed American Institution

Introduction

I have spent twenty-five years of my life as an enthusiastic member of medical academe, and my own career was largely shaped by this experience. I learned my trade as a clinician within the walls of two medical centers and later had the opportunity to acquire research skills and develop a good-sized research unit in one of them. I have the privilege of chairing a department of medicine in yet another and the joy of working with almost 300 young men and women doctors during their formative residency training period within that department. I was the dean of a fine academic medical center during the challenging period of the late 1960s and early 1970s when that institution and many others were taking on all kinds of new and difficult responsibilities. From these experiences I came to feel that I knew academic medical centers,* their strengths and their weaknesses, quite well. While it was clear that they were under increasing stress, so were many other institutions. I felt that they were making very significant contributions to our society and would work their way out of the problems that were buffeting them on all sides.

I now occupy a different vantage point, from which I can look at the academic medical center with somewhat more detachment.

*Throughout this section I have used the term "academic medical center" to describe the institution I am examining. As I employ the term, in its most simple form, the academic medical center includes a medical school and its teaching hospital. Obviously, most academic medical centers now contain a number of other important units. They may include schools of public health, dentistry, nursing, allied health professions, and an array of affiliated hospitals, outreach clinics, and other institutions that deliver actual medical services to people. However, it is the basic coupling of the educational mission of training doctors and a service mission that characterizes the institutions I am discussing.

Dr. Rufus Miles, former assistant secretary of HEW, once said, "Where you stand on an issue depends on where you sit," and I think that applies to me. After six years in the foundation world, with much of my foundation's activities focused on helping academic medical centers adapt to a new climate, I now can better recognize certain forces impinging on academic medical centers that I saw only dimly from the inside. This different perspective has given me a sharper awareness of the enormous external pressures under which academic medical centers are attempting to operate, and I am worried about them.

During the past decade, an unusual symbiotic relationship which has linked government and academic medical centers in a highly productive venture, has begun to come apart. This special partnership gradually evolved in the years immediately following World War II and reached full flower during the mid-1960s. The relationship developed because both parties shared certain concerns about medical matters and each had something to offer the other. Mutual interests included a desire to increase our national capacity to conduct high quality biomedical research, to improve and upgrade the knowledge base and skills of new physicians, to strengthen the training of medical specialists, to better regionalize sophisticated high technology services in tertiary care hospitals, and to give higher quality services to those unable to pay for private medical care.

This relationship was important because both government and the academic medical centers gained much from the arrangement. In it, government got well acquainted with a growing group of institutions that housed top academic medical talent. The physicians and scientists who made up the faculties of academic medical centers could advise those in government on major scientific and medical issues that confronted the nation and could often initiate new programs of interest to both parties that could not be launched by the public sector. This symbiosis permitted swifter responses to national mandates than would have been possible by either party alone. It also allowed government to better accomplish some other public sector tasks like training physicians for the developing countries, strengthening the staffing of veterans hospitals, putting well-qualified specialists in community hospitals, developing neighborhood health centers in poverty areas. Thus, it helped this country to work imaginatively on a number of other issues of national importance that were peripheral to the central thrust of medical academe. It gave those in positions of national responsibility entree to a group of intelligent, committed, and reasonably friendly colleagues in what then appeared to government to be the hostile climate of the private practice of medicine.

University medical centers also gained much from the relationship. They were able to move swiftly to build a strong biomedical research capacity and a broader range of high quality specialty training programs of international distinction and to greatly strengthen medical education in the process. Via the back door of government research funding, teaching medical centers were also able to increase their medical services to low income people, particularly those with serious complex illnesses where their high technology services excelled—to the benefit of all concerned.

But now things are going awry, and the interaction between those in government and those in medical academe is increasingly confrontational. From the federal viewpoint, academic medical centers, formerly believed to be a part of the solution, are now being viewed as the cause of the problem. Medical school deans who used to be asked to Washington for advice are now called there to be lectured on how unresponsive their institutions are to national concerns. For those responsible for academic medical centers, their enormous efforts to help solve national problems in medical care now seem to be forgotten, ignored, or denigrated by those in the federal health establishment. Thus, academic medical centers often feel that government is now using its spending power to prescribe educational policies in medical schools in ways that are unfair and shortsighted. It now seems that government feels that it should have a say in who should be admitted, the size of classes, the nature of the curriculum, and the kinds of careers students should pursue. This confrontation, and the involvement of government in the inner workings of medical schools, coupled with the increasing regulation of the teaching hospitals that academic centers run, has made many feel that these institutions are beginning to be bent and distorted in ways that may be a disservice to us all. Thus, government and academic medical centers currently seem on a course, not fully of their own making, that is increasingly adversarial.[1] The cessation of federal help to the Association of American Medical Colleges after a decade of support and the recent refusal of four major universities to accept critically needed capitation funds for medical education because of the unacceptable strings attached shows how far this confrontation has gone.[2] In the final analysis, this is a confrontation that academic medical centers cannot win, but alas, neither can government. In the end, society may be a loser, for these complex institutions—academic medical centers—have in the main served us well.

Failure to resolve this confrontation would be tragic. My own reading of history suggests that, over the long haul, society benefits richly from having its social and educational institutions pursue their destiny with considerable autonomy and flexibility. We have,

as a nation, always prided ourselves on the independence of education from government even in the closest of working partnerships
between the public and private sectors. We seem at hazard, however,
of forgetting this basic American ground rule insofar as it applies to
the training of physicians and to the administration of the centers
in which this training takes place. It seems ironic that as the nation
is moving away from regulation in so many areas, it is coming to em-
brace it in the field of medical education and practice. Looking back
at the history of American medicine, I simply do not believe that we
would have come as far had government been calling the tune in, say,
the 1920s. Would pediatrics have emerged as a specialty? Would we
have geneticists or perinatologists? Would tissue culture permitting
the development of a polio vaccine have evolved? Would we know
the biologic functions of cyclic AMP? I do not know, but I doubt if
some of the apparently aimless meanderings of medical science that
have led to spectacular advances in medicine would have been high
on a governmental priority list. Government marches to a different,
more pragmatic, drummer, and rightly so.

There has been much written about the shortcomings of academic
medical centers. I have contributed to that literature. But almost
nowhere have I seen any analysis of how they got the way they are
or how the evolution of American society and pressures on the body
politic have brought powerful unexpected forces into play that have,
and are, putting enormous and perhaps unwarranted pressures on our
academic medical centers. These institutions are now faced with
many problems that they simply cannot solve themselves, and much
of this seems to be occurring because neither party, academe or
government, fully hears or understands the other. As Dr. Walsh
McDermott has characterized the situation, "For most problems in
public policy and for all that are science-related, we must form our
judgments from hearing an argument between those whose comprehension of the question may be grossly warped because they do
not know the subject from the inside and those who perceptions may
be grossly warped because they *do* know it from the inside."[3]

I have lived in both the internal and external world of medical
academe. Though my long career as a faculty member may still
classify me as an "insider," I want to try here to interpret one group
to the other in a reasonably even-handed way. In my judgment,
academic medical centers cannot genuinely fulfill their very special
role in our society unless the public and the government understand just what created their current difficulties and assist them more
imaginatively. Conversely, medical center inhabitants need to understand better the concerns of society and to grapple with certain

problems more aggressively if the independence of academic medicine is to be preserved. For despite their central role in the order of medical things and their recognized achievements, academic medical centers currently occupy a difficult and troubled place on the American scene. They are at present beset on all sides, and the list of those groups that are unhappy or dissatisfied with their performance, or what they are about, is startlingly long.

1. State legislatures and governors are unhappy with academic medical centers because of their seemingly inexhaustable requirements for additional funds and the fact that their graduates rarely seem to end up practicing in local communities needing doctors, which prompted these legislatures to launch their state medical schools in the first place.
2. The federal sector has been increasingly disturbed by the apparent inability of academic medical centers to turn out enough physicians of the types that seem to be needed to care for the commonplace medical problems of the American population and by the requirements of these centers for vastly more federal funds than anticipated.
3. Academic Medical centers are a source of alternating pride and dismay to their parent universities. Faculty members of other divisions within the university watch the medical school, with its much generous faculty to student ratios and much higher salaries, turn out one-tenth to one-hundreth as many graduates as they do while hungrily gobbling up sometimes as much as one-half of the university's budget in the process.
4. Residents of the local communities and city neighborhoods in which these centers are located decry their relentless acquisition of property; areas occupied by private homes, playgrounds, small businesses and the like, are brought up by medical schools for parking, laboratories, or teaching facilities. City and town governments bemoan the attendant loss of taxable property.
5. Citizens living within the catchment areas of academic medical centers who turn for care to their emergency rooms or out-patient departments are distressed by the long waits they must endure, the impersonal care they receive from medical center personnel, and the appalling costs of that care, particularly if they are admitted to the academic medical center hospital.
6. The progeny of academic medical centers—the private physicians who graduate from them to practice outside the academic institution—have a complex love-hate relationship with them. They display their school diplomas in their offices, but berate them for

their enormous increases in size, their liberal leanings, their lack of understanding of the demands of practice, their failure to respond to practitioners' needs for continuing education, and their intrusion into community hospitals, thereby competing for the same patients who are the private practitioner's livelihood.

7. House staff who are receiving training within their walls frequently complain about being worked too hard, being paid too little, and not receiving adequate supervision by faculty; some also cite the failure of the institution to properly serve the poor who use it.

8. Even medical students—the young men and women who sacrificed, struggled, and bent heaven and earth to be admitted to academic medical centers—are often cross with them. They complain about the lack of relevance of what they are taught, the focus of faculty on research rather than on education, the denigration of the generalist careers they aspired to when they entered by their primarily specialist faculty, and the mountainous rises in their tuitions.

This is indeed a puzzling, schizophrenic situation, and rational human beings might ask. What in heaven's name has happened? Why do academic centers look like they do and behave as they do? Those who populate and run academic medical centers seem in the main to be intelligent people with lofty hopes of bettering the health of mankind and creating new tools with which to achieve that goal. How is it, then, that academic medical centers, which appear to be of such critical importance to the whole system of American medicine, seem to have so few friends? Are they worth saving, or have they outlived their usefulness?

My answer is predictable. I believe that they are worth saving. As a matter of fact, I believe they are, to use an overused expression, a unique American institution. In this section, I will try to characterize and quantify what they do (Chapter 5), to describe some of the external pressures under which they are now operating (Chapter 6), and to offer some suggestions for improving their lot (Chapter 7).

Chapter 5

Academic Medical Centers
as Special Institutions

These university appendages—the academic medical centers—occupy a central position in our whole complex American health care enterprise. They train most of the doctors and many of the other health professionals who work in our system of medical care. They generate most of the new medical knowledge that is being brought to bear on disease. Further—and it is this facet of their operations that brings them into daily interface with the public and the political world—they staff and operate the major high technology hospitals that are the pacesetters for medical practice throughout our country.

Their role in teaching, research, and patient care has made them big businesses. Some have physical plants valued in excess of a quarter of a billion dollars. It now costs between $100 and $200 million to launch a new one,[1] and, as shown in Table 5-1, the annual operating budget of major centers can exceed $100 million. Collectively, the 120 academic medical centers and their hospitals employ over a quarter of a million people and operate at a cost in excess of $12.5 billion a year.[2] Another significant indicator of the importance of academic medical centers is the amount and kind of care their hospitals provide. In 1976, almost 30 percent of the visits made to hospitals by American people seeking help for medical problems were to the emergency rooms and outpatient clinics of medical-school-affiliated hospitals.[3] In general, some of the best-trained doctors are connected with these hospitals, and anything new in diagnosis or management is apt to be found there first. People seeking the ultimate in care frequently ask to be admitted to an academic center hospital.

Table 5-1. Annual Operating Costs of Selected Academic Medical Centers (millions of dollars)

	1954–1955		1972–1973		1975–1976	
	Medical School Only*+	Major Teaching Hospital	Medical School Only*	Major Teaching Hospital	Medical School Only*	Major Teaching Hospital
Johns Hopkins University School of Medicine/The Johns Hopkins Hospital	$2.3	$ 9.464	$50.17	$56.42	$64.89	$ 76.007
Columbia University College of Physicians and Surgeons/Presbyterian Hospital	3.0	16.727	65.99	79.249	84.87	109.600
The Pritzker School of Medicine/University of Chicago Hospital	2.0	6.578	44.09	40.366	54.98	58.189
University of Pennsylvania School of Medicine/University of Pennsylvania Hospital	2.2	10.020	47.32	63.193	57.00	88.026
College of Medicine and Dentistry of New Jersey (Newark)/Martland Hospital	NA	NA	18.15	NA	23.48	30.525
Cornell University Medical College/The New York Hospital	1.1	14.768	23.27	71.617	40.90	98.923

Sources: Association of American Medical Colleges Liaison Committee Annual Questionnaire; *American Hospital Association Guide to the Health Care Field*, American Hospital Assoc., Chicago, Ill., 1955, 1973, 1976 ed.

*Teaching and research costs only.
+Medical school costs for 1954–1955 are estimates.

The large role that the hospital part of the medical center plays in delivering an actual service makes the medical school quite a different creature of the university than other graduate professional schools. All professional schools have some special obligations to the public they serve. The public trust requires that lawyers, engineers, and doctors be "credentialed" for the protection of those who depend upon them, but the university's responsibility stops there. There are some members of medical academe who argue that medical schools should also be allowed a more detached role, more parallel to other graduate schools. Their argument runs that law schools do not have responsibilities for the design or conduct of the legal system, schools of business do not determine the operation of the financial marketplace, and schools of engineering are not held accountable for the transportation system. Why then should medical schools have to bear so much responsibility for the medical care system?

Part of the answer to this question lies in the distinction between a medical school and a medical center. Columbia University does not have affiliations with any law firms, brokerage houses, or architectural firms. It does however, have an affiliation with Presbyterian Hospital—and many other hospitals and clinics as well. Consequently, the academic medical center has a much bigger piece of the action than other professional schools in a university. The new advances, the new technologies that shape practice, emerge from there. Whereas the Supreme Court, an institution totally removed from academe, serves as the ultimate authority for the legal profession, it is the teaching hospitals that serve as the last court of appeals for the medical profession. They are the ultimate resource for the diagnosis and management of those who are seriously ill, and the university connection with the hospital is, to date, our best form of "quality assurance."

While this situation creates considerable stresses, it also has some powerful strengths. The unique nature of this interesting arrangement was well described by Dr. Walsh McDermott in an address given almost fifteen years ago.

In a sense, the whole idea of a university medical center is preposterous, for it consists of turning over something really important—our families' health or life—to the management of a bunch of college professors. You may demure, "Well, the proposition is not really quite that raw, for everybody knows that medical professors are not really professors. They get haircuts with reasonable frequency, the coat and pants usually match, sometimes there is even a vest, they are obviously very clumsy with a pipe as they try pathetically to give up cigarettes—they mostly commute from Westchester, and a fair number can even be counted on to vote Republican, or at least to vote Republican when it 'really counts'." In short, they are not academic types at all, but practical fellows such as me and thee, well-skilled in the arts of meeting the payroll.

All this is true—in the sense that any stereotype has truth—but let us not delude ourselves—they are university professors, too—in all of the important, age-old university traditions. It is this incredible alloy of the creative intellectual, and the utterly practical, that is the hallmark of our great medical centers. Nowhere else in our society are these two great forces harnessed with such intimacy and such immediacy for the creation of a product—in this case, our better health.[4]

It is, I believe, the melding of the intellectual nature of scientific exploration with the intensely pragmatic demands of caring for the sick that has made academic medical centers such a vital force in our society. To my knowledge we have no other institution that plays this kind of role. The combination of service and research in an educational milieu tends to evoke the best that people have to give. It is precious and worth maintaining.

※ *Chapter 6*

Current Problems of Academic Medical Centers

As I stated earlier, the special nature of the academic medical center gives it not only its strengths but also special vulnerability. The chief pressures that academic medical centers are currently under stem from a number of factors—problems of location and size, a lack of coordination between government and organized medicine, a conflict between the need for generalists and the academic medical centers' specialist orientation, and the increasing "medicalization" of social problems. Let me expand on each of these.

THE PROBLEM OF GEOGRAPHIC LOCATION

Of the 120 academic medical centers in the United States, 32, or more than one-quarter of them, including some of the most prestigious ones, sit squarely in the midst of our largest, most troubled inner cities. Indeed, over half—sixty-one—are in the forty largest cities.[1] Herein lies a problem.

The older academic medical centers, or more precisely, the teaching hospitals of those centers, were built in the more heavily populated sections of the large cities for entirely sensible reasons—indeed, for laudable and humane ones. These early medical centers emerged with a dual purpose. They were primarily established as hospitals to treat the sick poor and patients who were referred to them, and they coupled this with the training of the next generation of physicians by letting them participate in that care. A broader educational goal was gradually grafted upon this primary mission, but it has been only within the past forty-five years that research has become a major component of academic medical centers. To give hospital care to those without it or to those with special problems was their initial raison d'etre. The heavily populated sections of our major cities were where the largest concentration of people with the greatest medical needs resided. Teaching hospitals located where the action was.

The areas of major cities in which these hospitals were established were very different then than they are now. While they contained some who were poor, they were largely middle and lower income communities. Because cities were much smaller and, more important, more heterogeneous, poor families often lived on the same block or around the corner from middle class families or even quite well to do families. The local shopkeeper, lawyer, grocer, clergyman, dentist, and policeman lived there, too. The doctors giving general ambulatory care had their offices in the areas surrounding the medical center. All of these wage earners formed a stablizing island of people who had a real stake in their own neighborhood. They maintained it and were constantly striving to improve it. But for all kinds of complex reasons, these responsible "people islands" have largely disappeared from the areas of our cities where medical centers are located.

First came the exodus of all those able to obtain better housing outside the inner city. With the departure of many wage earners, went the banks, the retail stores, and the grocery stores. Their disappearance left vast areas of inner cities without businesses, adequate transportation, police or fire protection, street lights, garbage collection, places for recreation, and other social structures that create a sense of community. Physicians in private practice inevitably followed the suburban-bound working class. As an example, in 1940, Baltimore had 950 physicians providing care to 850,000 residents, roughly 112 physicians per 100,000 people; these physicians were fairly evenly distributed, and most provided primary care. By 1971, the number of physicians practicing in the city had dwindled to 300, while the city had grown to 920,000 people, cutting the doctor to population ratio to 33 per 100,000.[2] In the core of the city, its poorest sections, the ratio was even worse.

Coupled with these changes was a marked shift in the racial mix of the inner city population in the largest cities. Between 1950 and 1970, the white population of all central cities in the United States increased by less than 10 percent. In this same time period, the black population rose rapidly in the central cities, increasing by 98 percent. This differential growth rate was even more pronounced in the forty largest U.S. cities, which experienced a net decrease of more than one million whites and a 111 percent increase in the black population during that twenty year period.[3] This increase was initially caused by a massive migration of poor rural Southern blacks to major cities. Although this migration had been anticipated, it occurred much more rapidly than anyone had expected. Thus, while a demographer predicted in 1958 that "within 30 years Negroes will constitute 25 to 50 percent of the total population in [the central cities of] at least 10 of the 14 largest [metropolitan areas],"[4] within two years this had become a fact.[5] Along with this came an influx, chiefly to the coastal cities, both east and west, of poor Spanish-speaking people from the Carribean and Mexico. With these changes, our inner cities have come to be desolate ghettos for poor nonwhites. Indeed, in certain areas they resemble the firebombed central cities of Europe during World War II. Within them, and often dominating the landscape, remains one major institution—the academic medical center.

Obviously, medical centers did not create the present problems of the cities. John Hopkins did not cause or encourage the progressive decline of East Baltimore. Columbia did not generate the events that had led to West Harlem. The University of Pennsylvania was not responsible for the dissolution of inner Philadelphia. Indeed, medical centers have been one of the few stablizing institutions remaining in our tortured inner cities. But the decision of these medical centers to "stay with it" has had profound undesirable side effects for them.

The departure of physicians and their convenient offices and the loss of other social services that help people cope left those in the central cities with nowhere to go for care except the one remaining facility—the medical center. The demands on these hospitals by people needing ambulatory care began to mount rapidly. Emergency rooms became the substitute for the local physician and were mountainously overtaxed. Outpatient departments designed for modest ambulatory care practices began to be overwhelmed by the enormous patient population looking to them for all medical services. The magnitude of this shift is dramatically portrayed in Table 6-1. Over the twenty year period between 1956 and 1975, the number of visits to the outpatient services of teaching hospitals rose by over 700 percent. In addition, inner city residents also began to look to the academic medical center, one of the few sources of employment remaining in the area, for jobs, and the centers thus found themselves with another responsibility not in their original mandate.

To make matters worse, the collapse of or failure to upgrade inner city transportation systems, the increasing personal hazards of venturing into the area around inner city medical centers, and the burgeoning of attractive suburban hospitals with plenty of parking spaces, caused a falloff in referrals of patients of higher incomes to

Table 6-1.   Ambulatory Visits in the United States, 1956 and 1975

visits in millions)

	1956	1975
Total ambulatory visits	700.0	1042.5
Visits to all hospitals	66.0	254.8
Visits to all hospitals as percent of total visits	9.4	24.4
Visits to all teaching hospitals	9.9	72.7
Visits to teaching hospitals as percent of all visits to hospitals	15.0	29.0

Source: Estimates prepared by John E. Craig of the Health Policy Research Group, Georgetown University, using National Center for Health Statistics and American Hospital Association Annual Survey data.

the academic medical centers. Thus, the centers were left with vastly more patients than they could adequately manage, many of them unable to pay for the services they needed; the inexorably rising costs of the whole academic enterprise; and a rapidly declining population of patients from higher income groups with the kinds of complex problems teaching centers were best able to manage, who could also help foot the bill.

If all this was happening, why did the academic centers reamin in the inner cities? Certainly other institutions saw the handwriting on the wall. Department stores, supermarkets, banks, and other institutions began early on to hedge their bets and to develop new branches in shopping malls and in the suburban periphery of the cities. Where were the medical planners and futurologists as these events began to move so relentlessly?

Again, the answers are complex. First, though often doubted by today's cynical society, those who work in or govern over academic medical centers are generally a rather idealistic lot. Most who opted for faculty or administrative positions in our academic centers in the 1930s, 1940s, and 1950s made a conscious decision to work for salaries lower than what they could command in private practice, in order to devote their careers to teaching, to doing research, and, last but not least, to delivering sophisticated hospital care to patients without regard to their ability to pay.

To become a member of medical academe at that time was a decision with very significant personal economic consequences. Academic faculty positions during those decades had salaries ranging from one-tenth to one-third of what one could make in private practice. (This is no longer true.) This of itself meant a self-selected group who put these other callings well above personal recompense. Obviously, many in the private practice of medicine had and still have similar priorities, but the point is that this fact of life tended to make most members of academe of similar persuasion and attitudes in this regard. They wished their medical centers to be located precisely where they are—in the centers of population groups who would, in exchange for expert medical services, permit medical students and house staff to participate in their care so that they in turn could become knowledgeable physicians. These faculty did not consider the ability of patients to pay their concern. On the contrary, they felt that their clinical teaching services might suffer if there were a decrease in the admission of poor or indigent patients.

In addition, members of medical academe were reluctant to compete with their own graduates and with the system of private medical care. Wishing to have time for research and teaching and study, few academic clinicians desired to have large private practices. They were comfortable caring for those not included in the private system of medical care and relying on referrals of patients with the most complex problems from their private colleagues to keep their special skills and high technology units functioning optimally. The central city location was an advantage in this regard. (Those who were pragmatic also realized that, if push really came to shove, academically oriented physicians might lose in any contest for patients if competing with well-organized private practices designed exclusively for patient care; certain academic health centers that have moved to the suburbs have learned that this can indeed be the case.)

It is, in the main, these members of the academic community, who graduated between, roughly, 1930 and 1960, who have shaped the attitudes of today's academic medical centers. One might properly argue that while their attitudes and splendid disregard for "bottom line" financing might characterize the faculty who populate the medical school and teaching hospital, surely the trustees of academic centers have different perceptions and better business sense. The answer to this is not so simple. Most trustees do come from business backgrounds and can readily see the extraordinary problems of trying to balance budgets of such an enterprise. But the governance of academic medical centers is not that of most organizations. Medical centers have few of the formal characteristics of industrial firms, and those who have tried to apply to medical centers some of the organizational strategies that have proved quite effective in business have not always had success.[6]

Among other things, distinguished medical faculty are a powerful lot and probably have more influence on trustees than would be the case in many other kinds of organizations. It is rare that trustees will act in opposition to a powerful professor of medicine who states that his teaching service will vanish if the institution moves, or to a strong-minded professor of surgery who insists that a new intensive care unit is critically needed to care for those (including the trustees) who come to the academic center for care.

Furthermore, many of the older academic medical centers were the result of an affiliation—often surprisingly vague—between a major hospital and a university, each with its separate board of trustees, priorities, and style. Thus Johns Hopkins, Columbia, Cornell, and Harvard, to mention just a few, all operate with at least two quite separate and distinct boards of trustees who must jointly reach agreement before any action can proceed.

Last, and perhaps most important, attitudes regarding the fiscal viability of academic medical centers vis-à-vis that of other kinds of enterprises has, until recently, been quite different. Bear in mind that most of the older teaching hospitals were private, voluntary, charitable institutions. By long custom, society, and particularly those who chose to serve as trustees of these institutions, expected to have to make up deficits from outside sources. They did not ask or expect the hospital to run a breakeven operation. Universities, including their medical schools, were viewed in much the same way.

The progressive decline of inner cities and the increasing dependence of a deprived population of medical centers for care and for jobs has made the situation yet more poignant and the charitable nature of the enterprise yet more compelling.

PROBLEMS CREATED BY THE SIZE OF ACADEMIC MEDICAL CENTERS

Compounding the problem of location is the present size of most American academic medical centers. The growth since World War II in the physical plants, in the numbers of personnel working in them, and in operating costs has been staggering. (Table 5-1, which shows the changes in operating costs of five medical centers since the mid-1950s, dramatically illustrates this.) With such growth has come a certain ponderousness. It is easier to turn a sixteen foot canoe than an aircraft carrier. The enormous expansion in the size of academic medical centers occurring since the late 1940s was also dictated to a significant degree by outside pressures. The demands for more and better scientific research, more health professionals, and a wider range of services, as well as the expansion of private and public insurance to pay for medical services, all contributed to this expansion.

The success of our scientific enterprises in World War II was most impressive. What infusions of money and a national mandate had done to produce new, sophisticated technologies in wartime were not lost on the American public. Some exciting biomedical advances had also taken place. At the end of the war, the opportunity to put more monies in socially oriented programs led to an understandable focus on medicine. The discovery of penicillin, refinements in anesthesia, remarkable developments in surgery, and other dramatic biomedical advances led the American public to feel that a significant flow of public dollars to support the expansion of medical research within academic medical centers was an important investment. The charge was, "Find answers to some of the pressing disease problems that trouble us," and public monies began to go to academic institutions in increasing amounts. In 1950, $73 million in federal funds was allotted for research; by 1975, more than forty times that amount, or $2.8 billion, was being spent for research in health and medical care.[7]

These large infusions of research monies led to a dramatic change in both the size and the character of academic medical centers. No longer were they simply to be places to teach medical students and the hospitals of last resort to care for those with complex and life-threatening illness. They also became the centers for new biological science. Faculties were rapidly expanded, and most of those recruited were selected on the basis of their research backgrounds and research contributions. Indeed, these new faculty were recruited primarily for work in the laboratory, not for patient care. The funds to support them were public dollars, and clinical work and, to a lesser extent, teaching were actively discouraged. Academic medical institutions acquiring research funds for new faculty salaries had to promise that the clinical activities and teaching duties of these faculty members would be minimal—less than 10 percent of their time was a common agreement—to be sure that virtually all their energies would be devoted to the development of new biomedical knowledge. The number of full-time faculty 300 percent—from 13,681 to 39,300—between 1962 and 1976.[8]

This increase in research faculty led to enormous new capital needs for space to house them, their laboratories, and their expensive scientific equipment. The kinds of scholarly research activities that were once centered in a very few special institutions like the Rockefeller Institute for Medical Research, or the Thorndike Laboratories became commonplace in most academic medical centers.

This development inevitably led in turn to marked increases in personnel requirements and the need for bigger and more expensive facilities in all other parts of the center. As research began to bear fruit, what could be done for patients began to be extended, and the complexities of the technologies needed to give such care required increasing numbers of people to operate the new equipment and to carry out the new procedures and therapies. There was a marked expansion in the number of house staff—the young men and women receiving postgraduate training through the supervised practice of medicine—and increasing numbers of personnel of all sorts were needed to support the expanded research and service functions. Whereas the Johns Hopkins Hospital employed 184 house staff to manage the 1,400 inpatient beds in 1950, by 1977 this had expanded to 442. Similarly, the hospital had 2,344 employees in 1955; by 1975 this had jumped to 4,364.[10] As shown in Table 6-2, similar increases in numbers of employees were occurring in other institutions.

Because of their inner city locations and their pressing needs for large numbers of employees, academic medical centers inevitably found that they were becoming one of the largest, if not the largest, employers of minimally trained people in the central cities. The

Table 6-2. Employment in Teaching Hospitals Owned, Operated, and/or Controlled by Academic Medical Centers, 1955 and 1975

	1955	*1975*
Academic medical center teaching hospitals*	83,854	259,858
VA hospitals+	49,006	91,332
The Johns Hopkins Hospital	2,344	4,364
The New York Hospital (Cornell)	2,649	5,335
Presbyterian Hospital (Columbia)	3,476	5,054
Martland Hospital (College of Medicine and Dentistry of New Jersey)	NA	1,675
University of Chicago Hospital	1,308	2,657

Sources: American Hospital Association Guide to the Health Care Field, 1955 and 1975 eds; *American Medical Association Directory of Approved Internships and Residencies,* 1955 and 1975 eds.

*Includes all owned hospitals and most of those operated or controlled by academic medical centers.

+Includes only those VA hospitals with major teaching programs.

kinds of jobs that needed doing led to the development of a huge semiskilled work force, and academic centers became major employers of blacks and women in the central cities.

Initially, this massive expansion in faculty, house staff, and support personnel did not cause serious financial problems for academic centers. The salaries that support staff were paid were traditionally very low. New house staff were added almost for free. The full-time faculty were paid modest salaries, and private practitioner physicians generously donated their time to train house staff and students and to supervise much of the patient care.

But in the 1960s this began to change. First, because of the increasing costs of hospital care, private insurance was rapidly expanding its market. To fill the gaps, public insurance programs—first Medicare and later Medicaid—were enacted, meaning that hospitals began to be recompensed for much of the care that had previously been given free. No longer so clearly "charitable institutions," hospitals began to be pressured to live up to minimum wage standards. Academic medical centers became a logical target for civil rights groups, and labor unions moved into the arena as well. The large size of the hospital workforce and their low wages made them a very visible and receptive group for labor unions seeking new members. Collective bargaining, even strikes—formerly unthinkable in hospitals—entered the picture, resulting in rapid and substantial increases in the salaries of hospital workers. As an example, whereas in 1960 the wages for hospital employees in Baltimore ranged from 60 to 68 percent of those paid in other industries, by 1969, they had jumped to 93 to 102 percent of the wages paid in other industries.[11] Similar changes in hospital wages were occurring nationwide.

At the same time, the young physicians who formed the resident staff also began to demand a living wage. Previously, young house staff doctors had been underpaid or not paid at all. In the 1960s, many residents were married and had families, a situation that had been uncommon prior to World War II. This group also began to receive significant salaries, and because their numbers had by this time become very large, this created another major expense for teaching hospitals. As an example, in 1949–1950, the 184 house officers receiving training at Johns Hopkins cost the institution approximately $55,000 in annual wages, an average annual salary of $290 per person. In 1977, the 442 house officers then employed received over $4.8 million in salaries, or better than $10,000 per person per year.[12]

As a final straw that threatened to break the academic medical center's financial back, the very research dollars that had permitted expansion in faculty ranks, coupled with new monies now received from insurance coverage, were used to substantially increase full-time faculty salaries. The gap between salaried physicians who worked within the medical center and those who practiced medicine outside narrowed considerably. And as private practitioners watched their salaried colleagues begin to make incomes approaching their own, and as they were displaced to less important teaching roles, these private physicians, formerly quite willing to donate their time, became less willing to do so, and either requested and received payment for their academic services or disappeared from the teaching scene to spend more time in remunerated pursuits.

Hospitals and academic health centers are labor-intensive—some 70 percent of their costs go to paying their personnel. The massive increase in numbers of personnel, the increasing expense of paying them, the enormous size of the physical plants, and the increasing expense of the high technology developed by academic centers made costs soar. It could not have been otherwise.

As a result of all of these changes, academic medical centers became saddled with the whole bewildering set of complex bureaucratic rules and constraints that we impose on large American institutions. A recent task force pointed out that 164 different regulatory agencies have some jurisdiction over hospitals in New York State. Some twenty-five separate agencies review admitting procedures, thirty-three are involved in protecting patient rights, and thirty-three agencies monitor patient safety![13] Similar constraints confront the academic centers in other states. Academic medical centers are now required to follow appropriate rules regarding wages, overtime, fringe benefits, and workmen's compensation. They must conduct ongoing sensitive, time-consuming negotiations with unions to prevent potential disruption of services. They must conform to local zoning and land use restrictions. They must adhere to governmental regulations regarding rates of overhead, methods for purchasing, hiring practices, affirmative action compliances, and construction of new facilities. They must answer to community planning boards, conform to standards for industrial safety and environmental protection, and so on.

This is a large order for a bunch of doctor-scholars. The governance of medical centers, stemming as it has from university origins and traditions, tends to be decentralized, ad hoc, vested in small committees, and focused on problems of scholarship, teaching, research, and the preservation of academic freedom. These governance mechanisms are ill-suited for dealing with the complex world of big business into which academic centers have been propelled.

PROBLEMS STEMMING FROM THE FAILURE OF PRIVATE MEDICINE AND GOVERNMENT TO FIX RESPONSIBILITIES FOR THE EQUITABLE DELIVERY OF MEDICAL SERVICES

A shifting national mood in the late 1960s led to a decision to put more monies into the delivery of medical services, and to lessen the escalation of support of biomedical research. In many ways, this was a logical, indeed inevitable, decision. The considerable fanfare surrounding some of the remarkable new biomedical discoveries that offered promise of decreasing human suffering had led to increasing public expectations about what medicine and medical science could do to improve the health and care of those who had footed the bill. However there was a widespread feeling that the fruits of biomedical science were not being promptly transmitted to the medical care side of things. (All subsequent studies have suggested that this is not the case, but the facts have not changed the perception.

At the same time, the soaring costs of medical care had been amortized across the board, increasing the expense not only of complicated medical procedures and highly skilled inpatient care, but also of more routine ambulatory care procedures. Thus, not only were many families, even those of middle income, finding the costs of major illness personally catastrophic, but many of the poor and near poor found themselves unable to afford even the most basic medical care.

An increase in private medical insurance helped to defray some of the personal costs of serious illness for most of the workforce, and Medicare and Medicaid were initiated to help with these costs for the elderly and the poor. By enacting these public programs, Congress was essentially echoing a change in national priorities—although federal support for biomedical research continued, the nation had decided to put new dollars into paying the personal costs of medical care.

Despite claims to the contrary, Medicare and Medicaid have helped considerably to alleviate the terrors of the expense of illness for those who are elderly or unable to pay for their care. They have done much good. However, the ground rules—the compromises that were required in order for this legislation to be passed—while greatly easing the problems of many community hospitals and enhancing the incomes of physicians, paradoxically intensified the plight of some academic medical centers.

One apparently innocuous sentence in the bill—a sentence viewed as vital by organized private medicine if it were to support these public programs—has led to real problems. HEW Secretary Cohen was able to launch Medicare, an experiment in insuring the costs of hospital care for the elderly, only by agreeing that it should in no way change traditional American mechanisms for the delivery of medical care. The fateful sentence: "Nothing in this title shall be construed to authorize any federal officer or employer to exercise any supervision or control over the practice of medicine or the manner in which medical services are provided, or over the selection, tenure, or compensation of any institution, agency, or person providing health services; or to exercise any supervision or control over the administration or operation of any institution, agency, or person."[14]

This made Medicare simply a financing mechanism for business as usual. It did not fix responsibilities for delivering care or encouraging experimentation in making services available to the elderly. It was silent on how care could be better distributed or gotten to those who were underserved. It permitted few new ventures in the way physicians and other health care practitioners were paid for their services. Actually, many academic physicians argued vigorously against the "business and usual" clause, insisting that it was both inflationary and restrictive, but their views did not prevail. There is a long-standing American tradition that government does not tamper with the private enterprise system, and with certain exceptions, this hands off policy has served us well. But the inception of public health insurance created some unforeseen events that prompted the federal sector to enter the medical scene in ways that were not expected.

It was anticipated that better financing of hospital costs would take voluntary hospitals out of their financial doldrums, and in the aggregate, this was indeed the case. While the total net income for nonprofit hospitals averged $112 million a year during the 5 years before the enactment of Medicare, it more than tripled, jumping to $359 million, between 1967 and 1969, immediately after the introduction of Medicare.[15]

Paradoxically, certain teaching hospitals appeared to fare as poorly as ever despite these infusions of funds. A personal vignette will serve as an example of why this occured.

As a professor of medicine at Vanderbilt University in the days prior to Medicare, I was distressed at the large numbers of sick people we had to turn from our doors because of their inability to pay. Thus, Medicare seemed an important step in the right direction. But the opposition of private physicians and organized medicine to this legislation was profound, and many of my practicing colleagues were unhappy about my support of it. While it eased our problems in admitting the elderly sick to our center, it intensified Vanderbilt's financial plight. In the years prior to Medicare, we had underwritten the costs of those unable to pay by vigorous use of the "Robin Hood" principle. By that I mean that those receiving private care in private accommodations were charged considerably more than their care actually cost in order to underwrite the cost of care for those unable to pay—an American custom of longstanding. When the money ran out, we simply could not admit indigent patients who could receive care elsewhere. But broad insurance coverage, including Medicare and Medicaid, largely eliminated both practices. The millionaire over sixty-five who occupied our hospital's most elegant accommodations had his bill paid by his insurance at about the same rates as that of the elderly ghetto tenant who was admitted to one of our wards. No longer could we adjust charges upward to obtain funds to pay for those who could not pay. There remained, however, many who were not covered by any form of insurance, and these patients were admitted as well. Thus, several years after the introduction of Medicaid, our university hospital seemed yet deeper in the red, while my practicing friends who had so opposed the legislation were finding their incomes considerably enhanced.

To return to my general thesis: Medicare cast the die. Those designing the legislation made the decision that they would pay costs but would in no way tamper with the private practice of medicine or with the problems of the distribution of medical care. As costs began to escalate, so did the anger, distress, and frustration of those in government who, in developing the legislation, had grossly underestimated its costs. As shown in Figure 6–1, the magnitude of these costs to the federal purse and the speed of their escalation were indeed remarkable following the enactment of Medicaid. In 1950, federal dollars spent on patient care averaged $6.38 per person. In 1966, sixteen years later, they had risen to only $16.83. But with public insurance the per person cost shot to $37.13 in 1967, $64.61 in 1970, and $131.92 in 1975.[16]

Governmental concern about costs caused officials to look at public insurance more carefully. Even if the costs could not be controlled, it was thought that at least the distribution of care could be made more equitable. Possible leverage points that might get care better distributed were sought. The practicing sector had, of course, been ruled out, so where else could pressures be applied? Academic medical centers seemed a reasonable target. They were by this time consuming substantial sums from the federal till. They were viewed as public or quasi-public institutions. And they were the villains

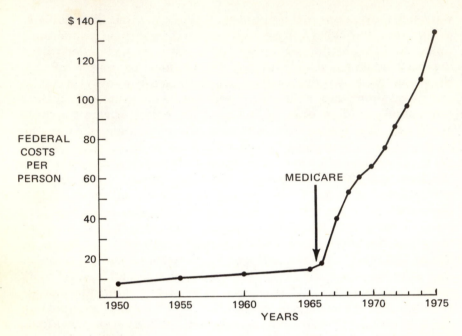

Source: Majorie Smith Mueller and Robert M. Gibson, "National Health Expenditures, Fiscal Year 1975," *Social Bulletin* 39, no. 2 (February 1976): Table 6.

FIGURE 6-1. Federal Expenditures for Personal Health Care, 1950–1975

who were responsible for having created all those expensive specialist physicians in the first place. What could be done to make them more responsive to public needs?

Now bear in mind that academic centers, while playing an important role in the care of the seriously ill, were at the time, only minor participants in the care of everyday sickness. Private physicians, practicing alone or in groups, were giving, and continue to give, the bulk of medical care received by our population—and this is the way both doctors and patients have wished it to be. But the failure of government and the private medical sector to arrive at some mutually agreed upon ways of distributing medical care led to the considerable power and persuasion of government being directed at academic medical centers to correct the imbalances. In an effort to cope with some of the areas not being addressed by the private system, academic centers were pressured to take on a bewildering array of new tasks. During the last decade, they have been asked to assume responsibilities for staffing and/or operating other public hospitals and neighborhood health centers; to develop rural out-reach clinics; to take on professional responsibilities for VA hospitals, including the recruitment of house staff to operate them; to make recommendations on medical care in prisons; to develop drug and alcohol abuse programs for the central cities; and much else.

Clearly these activities are not part of the traditional academic enterprise, and although I argued earlier that academic medical centers have more responsibilities for what is out there than other graduate schools, they should by no means be regarded as the only players—or, indeed, even the most important players—on the team in the delivery of medical care. The number of people in the health game, the small size of each unit within it, and the relatively small piece of the action directed by the academic center were not clearly recognized by government when it drafted medical academe to do its trouble shooting. Most governmental pressures of either a jawboning or a regulatory nature had previously been directed at industry. Here government was used to dealing with relatively few major films, knowing that if they could be brought in line, they controlled so much of the action that other smaller groups would follow. The 200 top manufacturing firms in the United States employ a third of the total work force in that sector and are responsible for 43 percent of the expenditures. The health care industry is of a very different nature, however. It is indeed a cottage industry, 95 percent of its units employing fewer than twenty people. In contrast to manufacturing, the 200 largest health care institution contain only 11 percent of all health care workers and account for only 8 percent of the expenditures.[17] Put quite simply, academic centers, despite their eminence are bit players in the total scene. Placing so many demands on them during a time of rapidly changing medical knowledge, increasing demands for health professionals, escalating costs, and dwindling endowments has grossly overloaded them in ways that seem both unfair and unrealistic.

THE PRESSURES OF SERVICE AND THE DISTORTION OF RESIDENCY TRAINING

One significant source of tension between government and academic medical institutions is the latter's apparent disregard for the kinds of doctors needed—their focus on specialist and subspecialist training, and their seeming lack of interest in training young physicians for generalist careers. All evidence suggests that more general physicians—family practitioners, general internists, and pediatricians—

are needed in our medical care system. Until very recently, however, almost 85 percent of medical school graduates became specialists, and only 15 percent went into generalist careers. The historical reasons for this, while not defensible, are nevertheless relatively straight-forward.

First, the clinical education of medical students as it is currently designed is conducted almost exclusively within a medical center's teaching hospital. The kinds of medical problems encountered in general practice are simply not in evidence in this setting. In a classic article on the ecology of medical care, Dr. Kerr White and his colleagues pointed out that among a typical adult population of 1,000 persons, about 750 experience some "illness" during each month. Of these, 250 consult a physician, and 9 are admitted to a hospital. Five are referred to another physician, generally a specialist. Only one is admitted to a university hospital.[18] It is this distillate of medical problems that engages the student.

Second, because the role of the academic center has been that of a referral center, the faculty who interact with students are, almost without exception, specialists who are primarily concerned with the problems of tertiary care and research. It is these individuals with whom the students have major contact during their formative years. Inevitably, these faculty become models, and students tend to pattern their careers similarly, despite the fact that the overwhelming majority of them ultimately enter private practice, not academic pursuits.

Third, some faculty members have maintained, albeit unrealistically, that they are not primarily responsible for the postgraduate segment of medical education and training—the residency period from which the differentiated doctor finally emerges. This period has traditionally been viewed as the responsibility of the various licensing boards, specialty societies, and the hospitals.

But last, and most important, it was primarily service, not medical education, that shaped the house staff training programs that are offered by academic medical centers. As the strengths and capabilities of academic medical centers grew, so did the referrals of patients with complex diagnostic and therapeutic problems who required enormous numbers of man hours and scientific and technical expertise for their management. The large number of clinical faculty who were hired and paid to do biomedical research meant that these faculty were unable (or unwilling) to spend as much time as was needed on patient care. Thus, there was a steady increase in the number of house staff recruited to meet the enormous demands of twenty-four hour a day, 365 day a year hospital coverage. Teaching hospitals were not much engaged in generalist care. They relied on the practicing profession to handle these problems. They were responsible however, for developing and maintaining the very special and complex kinds of care needed by the patients referred to them. House staff training was designed to extend these services, and residents served as the eyes, ears, and arms of the clinical specialists.

One might logically ask why these institutions didn't simply add more full-time faculty with clinical interest to take care of these special service needs. The answer is twofold. First, such a move was not viewed with enthusiasm either by the private practice sector, who did not wish to see salaried faculty practicing much medicine, or by the full-time clinical faculty who joined the university in order that their time would not be toally consumed by patient care. Second, additional house staff didn't cost much. Traditionally, interns were given room, board, uniforms, and laundry. Period. As a first year resident, after an unsalaried internship, I received a monthly paycheck of $16.67—a salary of $200 a year. As already noted, however, payment of house staff has changed dramatically in the last two decades. Annual salaries for interns now average slmost $11,000, and third or fourth year residents may receive salaries of in excess of $15,000. Thus, the cost of sustaining a house staff, formerly a trivial expense, now adds a significant amount to the costs of hospital care in major academic institutions.

While academic centers are now attempting to train more generalists—indeed, they now have a tough federal mandate to do so—the shift is difficult. Present faculties are simply not trained for the task; the patients coming to the academic center are atypical and do not generally present the problems encountered by those in general practices; and new linkages to other care centers which would give students a realistic yet controlled environment in which to learn more about general care, have not yet been fully forged.

The focus on training specialists, to the exclusion of generalists, has had still another untoward effect on academic medical centers, one that now paradoxically threatens their continuing viability. During the 1950s and 1960s academic centers were turning out large numbers of remarkably well-trained superspecialists from long and rigorous residency training programs. Certain programs, notably those in subspecialty areas of surgery, required as much as six or more years of postgraduate training. At the same time, stimulated by the Hill-Burton legislation, the nation was building new community hospitals at a rapid rate. The production of large numbers of elegantly trained subspecialist physicians, coupled with rapid development of new hospitals, led to quite predictable results. As these young specialists left the hallowed halls of academe to use their hard won skills, they set up shop in these new hospitals and established highly sophisticated subspecialty units that duplicated those on which they had been trained in teaching centers. We can wonder about whether so many high technology units were necessary—it is hard to defend maintaining four or five open heart surgery units or several cobalt treatment centers in one city—but this has occurred. And because these community hospitals were often well financed, admitting patients who were able to pay their bills, while referring those unable to pay to the teaching centers, community hospitals began to take referral business away from academic centers.

Here is the scenario: An outstanding academic cardiac surgical program trains a number of fine young cardiac surgeons each year. They cannot be accommodated at the mother institution, so they turn to the modern, well-financed hospitals on the outskirts of town, where they establish their own units, equipped with the most recent (and most expensive) equipment. The number of patients requiring cardiac surgery who are referred to the academic center begins to dwindle. All of a sudden there are three or four competing programs, all of high cost, in business in the same city. Each is doing between one-quarter and one-third as many operations as experts deem necessary to keep the skills of the cardiac surgery team in top form. Mortality and morbidity rates are higher in each institution than they should be in one fully utilized unit. The academic center runs harder and harder just to stay in place. Thanks to its own training program, it is far less of a referral institution than in days of yore. It is a victim of its own success.

Figures on the kinds of patients now coming to academic centers bear out this trend. When I was a house officer at the Johns Hopkins Hospital in 1948, 70 percent of the patients admitted were referred from outside the Baltimore area, indeed often from abroad. Now 80 percent of the patients admitted come from a ten mile radius of Baltimore, while those that used to come from afar are cared for in hospitals closer to home.[19]

The following five points sum up the "Catch-22" kind of situation that has been created in academic medical centers.

1. Teaching hospitals, initially created to admit a broad array of patients so that new physicians could be trained, become increasingly places to send patients with serious or complex illnesses that required the most sophisticated high technology care. The academic centers relied on referrals of patients from physicians in general practice in order to fill their hospitals' beds.
2. As the demand for special services rose, there was an increasing expansion of the teaching hospitals. More and more house staff

were recruited to render the specialist care required by the kinds of patients admitted to the medical center, and these young doctors became specialists in turn. Generalist physicians were not trained, and fewer and fewer graduates went into general practice.

3. As private physicians in general practice in the area died or moved to outlying areas, they were not replaced. The demands on the medical center outpatient department and emergency room for general ambulatory care escalated markedly, sometimes almost overwhelming the academic center's capacity to cope.

4. To add insult to injury, the graduates of the medical center's own specialty training programs established themselves in burgeoning new hospitals and began caring for the kinds of patients previously referred to the academic center hospital, causing a decline in the occupancy rate of the parent teaching hospital.

5. Because of the glaring misfit between the kinds of physicians being produced and those deemed necessary to answer national needs, the need for more general care services in the areas served by the teaching hospitals, the poor distribution of services, and the alarming increases in costs, the federal sector has set in motion increasing regulation of academic medical centers—regulation of a kind usually assiduously avoided in American society.

In general, government has left higher education alone, feeling that its institutions are quite sensitive to the demands of the market place. But the cascading events just described led the government to quite a different decision about its relationship with academic medical centers.

PROBLEMS CREATED BY THE MEDICALIZATION OF SOCIAL PROBLEMS

Last on my list of powerful external forces creating problems for academic medical centers is the interesting shift in our national perceptions of what constitutes a "medical" problem. Professor Renee Fox has written a fascinating article on the "medicalization" of certain kinds of social problems in the United States.[20] It deserves careful reading by all who are concerned about medicine.

During the last decade, many problems that seem to have emerged in part in response to the stresses, strains, and shortfalls of modern society have been moved into the purview of medicine. The overuse of alcohol, addiction to drugs, problems of violence, child abuse, disorder previously labeled "behavioral," marital incompatability, sexual identity problems, certain behavior long considered criminal, compulsive overeating, even gambling—these and many other problems have now been "medicalized."

I do not judge this as necessarily bad. Viewing thse kinds of social pathology as "medical problems" permits people to be less judgmental about them and to consider how they might be approached more objectively. But clearly, many of these problems have roots in situations that are not currently susceptible to medical solutions. Unhappy home life, unemployment, poverty, social alienation, and many of the stresses of modern American life play a role in their origin.

Be that as it may, many people with these kinds of problems are now asking academic medical centers for help, and those working in academic centers are trying very hard to cope with them. Obviously, physicians in private medicine see their share of these problems, too, but I would venture to say that the most profound and difficult of these cases now engage considerable amounts of the time of those working in academic medical centers. Given the current state of knowledge, they are not very successful with them.

There are a number of reasons for the shifting of these kinds of social ailments onto the physician. It has stemmed in part from increasing public expectations of what modern medicine can do and in part from dissatisfaction with the other social institutions that have traditionally dealt with these problems. As our society has grown more open, more tolerant of individual differences, and less tied to the mores of the past, a number of social institutions have failed to keep up. Thus, for example, organized religion, which used to play a very important role in helping people set their personal compasses, has become a progressively less important force in American society. The rigid tenets of our major religions seem unsatisfactory or unacceptable to many today. (As an example, consider the discrepancy between the dictates of the Catholic church on birth control and the actual practices of Catholic women.) Organized religion has tended to try to avoid involvement with messy problems like drug abuse, rape, and child beating. Similarly, the legal system has grown increasingly ponderous, and each day's news catalogues many of its inabilities to cope with the distressing problems of our modern world. It would seem that, in an effort to broaden the options for solutions, we have dereligionized and decriminalized some problems by viewing them in a medical context. Despite its shortcomings, medicine is viewed as more impartial and adaptive than other social institutions and as more morally and politically "neutral" in its approach to problems of highly polarized emotional content.

But the medical community—and particularly academic medical centers—did not ask to have these problems laid at their doorstep. While they have been willing to lend a hand—as an example of this willingness, some medical schools have established new departments of sociomedical science—the fact is that the physicians who staff academic medical centers are intellectually and tempermentally often the least well equipped to handle them. The multifactorial nature of these problems and their deep roots in situations that lie outside the classic concepts of disease or deranged physiology mean that they are generally not solvable within the medical model. They have been moved to medicine by default, and in the inner cities, where such problems are concentrated, the medical center has in many instances seemed to be the only game in town.

The problems these ailments create for the academic medical centers are enormous. Vast amounts of time, energy, money, and time are devoted to dealing with people with tragic maladaptions to life. These individuals now represent a high percentage of those who populate ambulatory clinics. That serious medical problems result from many of these unsatisfactory ways of coping with life are undeniable, and the wards of academic medical center hospitals now demonstrate this very dramatically. As an example, over one-third of the patients now admitted to the ward services of the Johns Hopkins Hospital are hospitalized for medical problems resulting from the use of alcohol.[21] Another significant fraction are admitted because of misuse of drugs. Drug-or-alcohol-induced coma, cirrhosis, bleeding esophageal varices, aspiration pneumonia, serious self-inflicted infections from contaminated needles, and bacterial endocarditis, all rare in society at large, are diseases now commonly seen in inner city hospital teaching services.

WHERE DOES THIS LEAVE THE ACADEMIC MEDICAL CENTER?

These, then, are some of the forces, largely external, that have been shaping academic medical centers. Many are beyond their control. Obviously, many internal forces have also been at play, but these are beyond the scope of what I wished to address in this particular chapter, for I believe that it has been these external pressures that currently threaten the continuing viability of the academic medical center. In the best of all possible worlds, it is the creativity and the vision of those who work within academic institutions, taking their cues from society at large, that determine the success or failure of the venture. But for academic medical centers, pressures that have came largely from without are increasingly dictating their course and probably unwarrantedly distorting their character and interfering with their full effectiveness.

The list of problems that academic centers currently face is sobering.

1. Located in the inner cities, they are overwhelmed by mounting responsibilities for ambulatory care and are attempting to deal with many people with problems that medicine in general and physicians in particular cannot manage very well.
2. Hard pressed to maintain their very expensive, technically complex units for patient care while their role as major referral centers dwindles as a flock of well-trained graduates from their own training programs develops competing modern services in suburban hospitals.
3. Struggling to maintain the cadre of biomedical scientists and the precious research efforts that have taken almost forty years to build, a role they recognize as critical if medicine of the future is to be better than that of the present—a role now viewed with less enthusiasm that in the past by an impatient public.
4. Attempting to be responsive to governmental pressures to take on many new responsibilities—pressures properly directed at the profession of medicine as a whole but, due to American political philosophies and the use of public dollars, now directed almost exclusively at academic medical centers.
5. Carrying the costs of a large number of house staff who are devoting most of their time to coping with the enormous and atypical problems of a teaching hospital service—often at the expense of generalist orientation and experience.
6. Losing their financial shirts in the process.

This is a worrisome situation for the institutions that have played such a vital role in the development of medicine as we know it today and that, I believe, remain vital to our future. As a nation, we simply cannot do without the institutions that educate and train the majority of our country's physicians and most other health professionals. Despite their problems, they continue to be the leaders in developing new biomedical science, and they possess the most sophisticated know-how for dealing with complex, life-threatening illness. They remain very special institutions, and no other entity has emerged to take their place. Clearly they need and deserve help.

※   *Chapter 7*

What Might Be Done?

It should be apparent from what has gone before that academic centers alone cannot solve many of the problems that confront them today. Indeed, in their travails, one can see an intense distillate of some of the problems that plague American urban society at large in the 1970s. It will require broad changes in many sectors to move us toward solutions to them. There are, however, certain steps that academic medical centers and the society that supports them might take right now that might begin to strengthen and improve their current situation.

1. The Governance of Academic Medical Centers Needs Examination and Probable Restructuring

A myriad of important complex relationships with the outside world and how these are shaped, organized, and managed, as well as the balance between service and scholarly pursuits, will determine the character and future viability of our academic medical centers. Decisions about interactions with government, labor unions, community developmental efforts, and the size and nature of medical service responsibilities not central to teaching and research missions need the vision and talents of people quite different from those traditionally developed in academic settings.

Here my suggestions may be viewed as paradoxical. I have indicated that medical centers are grossly overloaded with demands not of their making. But in regard to the milieu in which they operate—their size, location, and service loads—simply their own self-interest demands that they become more intimately involved in working with other groups in society to improve relationships and the sectors of our cities where they live.

Obviously this is not a role for which physicians, particularly academic professors, are trained. Professors of medicine or surgery do what they do very well, and it is unlikely that much more can be demanded of them. They are not management experts, financiers, city planners, or labor relations experts, and they and their faculty have neither the aptitudes, the talent, nor the inclination to work on these problems. But while in times past academic health center personnel could view themselves as largely "out-of-towners," responsible only for the calibre of their professional work in their enclaves, circumstances make this no longer a tenable position. These institutions and those who staff them must now recognize their importance not only as a source of care, but as major employers of people, managers of large systems, and a potential force for general good in their area. It follows that those who lead major academic centers in urban areas should probably be selected for quite different characteristics and experience than heretofore. Those who have become the chief executives of academic medical centers have traditionally moved through the faculty ranks as biomedical scientists, physicians who have distinguished themselves in clinical research, and teachers of medical students, before assuming their present roles. They are primarily skilled health professionals, not sophisticated financiers or city planners. Is it not time to consider that the current problems of academic medical centers require leaders with quite different interests, skills, and backgrounds?

The urban medical center is now commonly the major industry in its particular sector of town. The reasons for building many of them in our central cities remain—indeed, are even more compelling than when they were built. The enormous capital investments in physical plants and the absence of other institutions that can give medical help to people who live in these areas leaves them virtually no alternative. The problem is obvious. Can anything be done to improve the climate or the locale so that they can function more effectively? Must not the senior executives and trustees of academic medical centers put more of their energies and talents to work on improving the area in which they live or to work cooperatively with those best equipped to do it? Clearly, other major industries have and would. Witness the efforts of Prudential Life Insurance Company to upgrade central Newark. Examine the remarkable rebirth of sections of inner Philadelphia or the Crown Center Development in Kansas City or the rebuilding of downtown central Baltimore. These developments were spearheaded by, planned, and implemented by the private sector institutions that live there. It was insurance companies, banks, retail merchants, and other large private enterprise industries that committed their time, effort, talents, and considerable amounts of their money to the process. Although the financial plight of academic medical centers will prevent them from making similar capital investments, they are in a position to command it from others.

To ask a physician or a trained hospital executive to do this kind of task does not make sense. They need to pilot the important and demanding affairs of science, teaching, and patient care. Clearly, these institutions must have such a "Mr. Inside." But perhaps a "Mr. Outside" should now play a more prominent role in meshing the institution more closely with its community and society. Why not select for this role the kinds of people who are trained for and enjoy this kind of activity? There are those who have large visions of what might be done to improve relationships between large institutions and government and our cities. They end up in positions as mayors, or governors, or chief executive officers of creative industries. Clearly, some people enjoy grappling with these kinds of difficult and complex problems.

I do not wish to be misunderstood here. I am not suggesting that academic medical centers be converted to social action agencies. The vital activities of those who work within the academic medical center must be protected and nurtured. Scientists must have the freedom and the opportunity to pursue their intellectual tasks. Teachers must be encouraged to teach. Doctors must care for patients. But I can visualize an administrative structure that places significant responsibility and authority for guiding the institution in the hands of a leader with a broad view of the role of the institution as a powerful community and national force, while instituting appropriate checks and balances to keep the academic enterprise intact. The leaders of such academic institutions must be more than experts in infectious disease or cardiology or medical education. Times have changed, and so must the governance of these large and important institutions.

Make no mistake, changing the governance of academic medical centers will require enormous effort, patience, and testing of new approaches. Placing real authority as well as responsibility in the hands of any centralized leadership will be stoutly resisted, and for understandable reasons. The governance of academic centers has developed along university lines. It is often ad hoc and consists of a series of coalitions that shift depending on the issue. It subserves the individual aspirations of researchers or clinical faculty quite well, but it falters badly when the institution is grappling with priorities or long-range goals. Harlan Cleveland, the former president of the University of Hawaii, addressed this situation well in an article entitled "How Do You Get Everyone in on the Act and Still Get Some Action"[1] I have discussed it peripherally in examining the dilemmas of medical deanships.[2]

The dilemma stems from the fact that people in medical centers carry out multiple functions simultaneously. Many of the rewards for superior performance are external to the institutions, and physicians tend to place more value on individual and peer group evaluations of their efforts than on institutional loyalty. Marvin Weisbord, a behavioral scientist skilled in organizational development, has written a thoughtful piece on the subject entitled "Why Organizational Development Hasn't Worked (So Far) in Medical Centers." In it, he points out that health professionals learn a vigorous scientific discipline as the "content" of their training. The process, he says, inculcates a value for autonomous decision-making, personal achievement, and the importance of improving their own performance rather than that of any institution.

> In consequence physicians identify much less with a specific institution and more with the culture of medical science. This constitutes a set of values, skills, and knowledge quite independent of any work setting. The rewards of major significance to them—respect, reputation—may come more from this larger arena than from their institutional affiliation.[3]

To reiterate, changes in governance that will permit more decisive institutional goals to be set and reached will not be easy, but I believe they are necessary.

2. Academic Medical Centers Should Prepare For Restricted Growth and Develop More Cooperative Linkages with Other Institutions

And what of the size and complexity of our academic centers? Here I would suggest "imaginative retrenchment." I have written elsewhere that academic medical centers must recognize that they probably now capture about all of the financial resources this country can afford and that they must begin to prepare for a "steady state" in which they can still become better, but probably not bigger.[4] Proper facilities for biomedical research, for teaching, and for other scholarly pursuits are critical to the future progress of medical science and the output of new health professionals. However, if we were to move to more regionalization of expensive technologies and services, academic medical centers could probably find ways of utilizing resources not necessarily within their walls. In cities where more than one academic medical center is located, the pooling of certain services seems a real prospect. For example, could not the Cornell and New York University Medical Centers, which are only two miles apart, share in certain ventures to mutual advantage?

Furthermore, if one views the future needs for medical care and projects trends in hospital bed requirements, the need for some reduction in the size of the in-hospital component of academic medical centers seems clear. The changing nature of illness patterns of Americans is reducing national requirements for hospital beds. This is a dramatic illustration of the forward march of American medicine. We used to require significant numbers of beds to take care of children with rheumatic fever and patients of all ages with bacterial pneumonia during the winter. Penicillin changed all that. Large orthopedic hospitals housed many children with chronic osteomyelitis and the crippling ravages of polio. Penicillin and the polio vaccines have virtually eliminated these problems. In older times there was a well-established ratio of beds to population allotted for the care of those with tuberculosis. Streptomycin and isoniazed rendered those figures meaningless. Psychopharmacologic agents have played a similar role in reducing the needs for beds for the mentally ill.

In 1876, America had 200 hospitals.[5] Between 1876 and 1950, hospitals were added to the American system at an average rate of almost ninety per year. During the period of 1950 and 1965, the rate declined to twenty-two per year. But as shown in Figure 7-1, since 1965 the number of hospitals has actually declined. Of even greater significance, despite a constant number of beds, the occupancy rates for American hospital beds have fallen steadily since 1950. It is clear that we are now an "overbedded" nation, and this contributes significantly to the high costs of medical care today. An Institute of Medicine study has recently recommended that we close 10 percent of these beds.[6] Thus, in planning for the future, academic health centers must recognize that their numbers of beds may decrease, despite an increasing number of students being trained. In planning for that steady state, they need to develop broader cooperative arrangements with other hospitals and to regionalize high cost facilities and services.

3. Government and Academic Medical Centers Must Collectively Reach Some Mutually Satisfactory Agreement on the Number and Kinds of Health Professionals Needed and Adjust Training Opportunities Accordingly

Projections regarding health manpower—the nature, number, and kinds of experience required by health professionals—is a highly

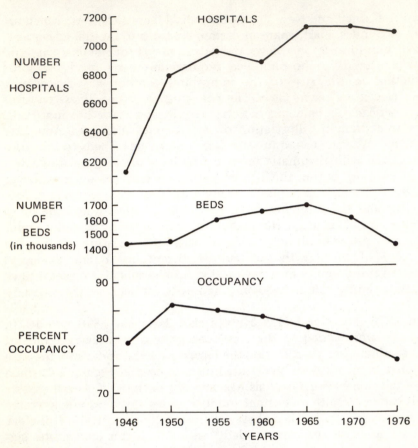

Source: Hospital Statistics, 1977 ed. (Chicago, Ill.: American Hospital Association, 1977), Table 1, p. 3.

FIGURE 7-1. Pattern of Growth in American Hospitals, 1946–1976

imperfect science. New technologic advances or changing social priorities can overnight render the best laid plans obsolete. Be that as it may, that adjustment in the nature of the clinical training offered by academic medical centers is needed to better respond to the medical care requirements of modern society is agreed by all. The postgraduate training programs developed in academic medical and teaching hospitals were in part responsible for the progressive disappearance of generalist physicians from the scene. It thus seems reasonable to suggest that academic medical centers have some responsibilities for working with government to correct the situation. Clearly, the time has come for academic centers to agree that house staff training programs designed simply to answer the massive and atypical service needs of the university teaching hospital fall short of fulfilling their responsibilities. House staff education and training must expose them to patients and problems that more accurately mirror the medical problems of society at large.

This does not mean that young physicians should be trained simply by having them work with the medical problems that are the daily fare of a generalist physician. Seeing large numbers of patients with viral upper respiratory infections or gastrointestinal upsets does not the physician make. The internist must readily separate congestive heart failure from pneumonia, or cirrhosis from constrictive pericarditis. Thus, disproportionate amounts of time must be spent in learning to recognize and treat those less common but potentially more serious problems. Hospital inpatient experience is the most efficient and effective way of developing these skills, and intense exposure to the unusual life-threatening illnesses that surface only infrequently will continue to require the lion's share of residency time. But broader acquaintance with and understanding of the common medical problems in practice is needed if we are to produce more broadly oriented generalist physicians.

To offer such experiences will require certain very significant adaptations by academic centers. To meet some of the high technology service needs of the university hospital may require hiring full-time trained physicians, not house staff, to deal with these problems. To give a more balanced education to those desiring generalist careers will require alliances with other health institutions that are coping with the kinds of illnesses that more adequately mirror those of the outside world.

Affiliations with ambulatory medical care units, nursing homes, daycare centers, school health systems, and the like could provide these broader educational opportunities. The participation of both doctors who educate and those being educated in care of people in these settings would have the added benefits of significantly upgrading the general medical care in those institutions. I would also guess that we will have to change the specialist-generalist ground rules if general medical care careers are to be made more attractive. My crystal ball tells me that specialists will need to become increasingly hospital-based, that the ground rules regarding referral to specialists will need to be honored more meticulously, and that the discrepancies between the incomes of generalists and specialists will have to be narrowed if we are to alter current career selections in medicine.

If academic institutions are to be asked to offer more out of hospital and ambulatory care experiences, more satisfactory mechanisms for financing ambulatory care and the costs of educating young physicians in ambulatory care settings will have to be developed. Although most Americans are insured either privately or publically for the cost of hospitalization, this is not the case for ambulatory care. That insurance coverage for out of hospital medical care is particularly inadequate for those in lower income groups was discussed in Chapter 3 and is well detailed in a recent article by Robert Blendon.[7]

We simply cannot ask academic institutions to make alliances with other institutions, expand their involvement in out of hospital care, or redesign ambulatory care training experiences without developing more satisfactory ways of paying for both the care and the educational endeavor as well. This is a problem for society in general. Its solution is out of the hands of the academic centers.

4. Government and Society Must Turn Their Attention to Strengthening of Institutions Other Than Medicine That Offer Human Support Services or Develop New Ones to Replace Those That Are Faltering

The medicalization of many social problems will continue to trouble us for many years. We simply do no know enough to deal with these problems effectively. We must, as a nation, continue to develop new knowledge about man as a social creature as well as a biologic one. Medicine will continue to struggle with these problems. But other social institutions that have traditionally been concerned with how people cope need to become more vigorously involved in developing that new knowledge. They need attention, encouragement, and money to do so. Religious groups and those responsible for legal services, psychologic aid, and other social services must also explore new approaches. We must find more satisfactory solutions to the social ills of violence, drug abuse, child neglect, and destructive behavior if American society, American cities, and the American lifestyle are to survive into the twenty-first century. Medicine can and should be a partner in working on these problems—but it cannot act alone. Some of the external pressures from government and society to find answers here should be directed more broadly.

5. Government and the Practicing Profession of Medicine Must Settle Their Differences and Decide How Care Can Be Better Distributed

Of absolutely critical importance, there must be much broader agreements on how these two major forces—government and private medicine—can together develop ways of supplying medical care with dignity and equity to those now underserved. The vast majority of our physicians—some 330,000 of them—are in the private practice of medicine. It seems appropriate for society to ask that these physicians as a group participate more fully in addressing the medical problems of those who do not now find their way into practitioners' offices. We are a large and diverse country, and Americans believe deeply in maintaining a pluralistic society. Clearly, the current problems we face in the delivery of modern medical care to all cannot be solved simply by government or legislative mandate. In my judgment, those who enter the medical profession owe a deep debt to the society they serve. Their education is to a significant degee subsidized by public dollars. Public funds have been used to develop the high technology equipment and services now in place in our private hospitals. Those hospitals and those who practice medicine within them are now subsidized by public funds. If medicine is to remain one of the bastions of individual enterprise in this country, those who practice it must work more cooperatively with government to collectively develop better solutions to deal with some of the inequities in our current system of medical care. Clearly academic medical centers should be involved, but how we will get health professionals and medical care to where they are not depends basically on cooperation between government and the private practice sector.

In this effort, the leadership of private medicine must be open to exploring ways of developing new institutional forms to get the job done. The solo practice of medicine has served us well. However, all evidence suggests that solo practice will not and cannot bring and maintain medical care in underserved poor urban and rural areas. The horse and buggy and the house call had their place, but both fail to meet the needs and demands of our modern world. New private arrangements that can attract health professionals to less desirable locales, link them with modern technologies, keep their skills current, and recompense them adequately must be developed—and the private sector working in partnership with government must roll up its sleeves and get about it.

The National Health Service Corps represents a government initiative to answer distributional problems. If it was understood by all entering medicine that they would be required to practice general medicine for a two year period in an underserved area before they could enter a specialty program, some of our maldistribution problems might be further lessened. But this falls short of the mark. It mandates an old solution to a modern problem. I believe more imagination and lasting solutions could be developed. The Robert Wood Johnson Community Hospital Program, which permits hospitals and their medical staffs to collectively develop cooperative arrangements to put services in place in underserved areas, linking these services to and supporting them from the hospital, is yet another and, I believe, more logical approach to a problem that will long be with us.

6. Last, the Cost Issue Must Be Faced Squarely By All Parties—Government, Academic Medical Centers, Hospitals, and the Practice Sector

At present, it is the cost issue, or more accurately the dizzying and relentless rise in medical care costs, that tears at the vitals of our whole medical care enterprise. It is escalating the confrontations between government and academe, government and private practice, hospitals and their medical staffs. Legislated programs and regulatory constraints—PSROs, HMOs, HSAs, hospital cost controls—all represent our current contorted and incomplete ways of grappling with this issue that so threatens the fabric of American medicine. In my judgment, they fall far short of the mark.

In the final analysis, costs—or ways to control them in ways all involved can live with—are a political problem. We must find ways of getting all parties to the table and of working through compromises on which we can all reach concensus. Academic medical centers are but one actor in this scenario, but they must play a cooperative role—and probably build more awareness of the cost implications of their acts into their graduates—the physicians of tomorrow. If academic institutions are to offer more out of hospital and ambulatory care experiences, we must develop more satisfactory mechanisms for financing ambulatory care and the costs of educating young physicians in ambulatory care settings. We simply cannot ask academic institutions to make alliances with other institutions, expand their involvement in out of hospital care, or redesign ambulatory care training experiences without being paid for it. This is a problem for society in general, but government and academe must understand each others problems in working on ways to manage the politically explosive issue of costs.

My recommendations for changes that might stabilize and strengthen academic centers and their relationships with government are not abstract. They stem from watching a number of academic institutions that are responding imaginatively and responsibly to the serious problems created by evolving circumstances. Some imaginative and vigorous leaders of academic medical centers are now addressing themselves to the problems of the quality of life outside as well as inside their institutions' walls. Some are reducing the number of inpatient beds in their hospitals and taking on new outreach medical care responsibilities for adjacent towns or establishing clinics in underserved areas. Many are forming new alliances with other institutions that deal with medical problems that are more representative of those ordinarily faced by people in our nation. Some are restructuring their postgraduate training programs to turn out more generalist-oriented physicians. Certain medical schools are incorporating new sciences such as medical epidemiology, sociomedical science, sociology, and behavioral sciences into the curriculum. Some governmental initiatives, like the National Health Service Corps, which places young physicians in medically underserved areas for a two year period, are directed at the maldistribution problem. But if ways cannot be found to solve the current "who struck whom" arguments that presently waste the energies of both parties, academic medical centers will be forced into a progressively more ambiguous and difficult situation which will make it unlikely that they can fulfill even society's most restrained hopes for them.

I hope some of these confrontational problems can be overcome, for academic medical centers are a precious national asset. Several years ago, Dr. Walsh McDermott put it this way in describing them.

> To me, this something special is that a medical center is one of the few places—perhaps the only place—where one can see the entire exciting process of the mind of man working at its best from start to finish.
>
> By the whole process, I mean the entire sequence involved: the birth of an idea; the establishment of its validity; the placing it in a usable concept; the teaching of it to others; the testing it for practical utility; the careful weighing of the moral and ethical questions that inevitably arise concerning its use; and its discriminating application for the benefit of a particular human being.
>
> Elsewhere in our society, the individual components of this glorious sequence are decentralized both in place and in time. But in a medical center, the sequence is in continuous operation and one can see it all at once.
>
> It is this, that makes the medical center more than a hospital, more than a college, or more than a research institute. And what is more this whole process which starts in the human mind and ultimately helps the mind or body of another, takes place in the physical setting in which the major events of life and witnessed everyday. The joyous birth of a child, the hope in the face of the patient who is recovering, the sadness of those about to be bereaved, and above all the great gallantry with which most people meet their death. These episodes of life and death are no mere backdrop for the intellectuality within the institution's walls—they are its major purpose.
>
> I am convinced that it is this fierce acceleration of the process, this ability to witness an idea from its start to its actual application for man's benefit, that gives the medical center its very special character.[8]

I can but simply second this. Medical centers do have a very special character, but their nature is being distorted by the demands being put on them. Both government and academic centers have to better understand each other and the circumstances that have led them into this situation. Society is not benefiting from the current adversarial positions. If the former more mutually supportive relationships can be reestablished, it seems likely that they can more satisfactorily accomplish their mission. This mission must be broader than some within these centers might wish it to be, yet narrower than what society now asks of them.

Part III

The Doctor's Dilemma:
The Physician as a Person

Introduction

In a thoughtful article outlining what would be needed if we were going to have an effective system for delivering general medical care to all people in this country, Dr. Walsh McDermott stated that one of the basic requirements for a well-trained physician was the ability to "identify, from innocent-appearing situations, those few that are potentially serious, and to provide properly for them:"[1]

This simple statement hides within it part of the enormous burden placed on physicians. Let me be more graphic. I still vividly remember participating as a third year medical student in the workup of a young student nurse in the emergency room of New York Hospital at 4 P.M. on a particular afternoon. Her story was simple. While on duty on a pediatric floor, she rather abruptly began to feel unwell. She had a chill, developed a headache, had a fever of 101°F, and "ached all over." She had vomited once. Examination by an excellent resident physician revealed little except a slightly inflamed throat. Her white blood cell count was not particularly elevated although it did show more immature polymorphonuclear leukocytes than normal. A urine specimen was unremarkable. A chest x-ray was clear. It was believed that she had the "flu," and she was reassured, given an aspirin, and sent to her dormitory to rest. At midnight she was returned to the emergency room by some of her classmates. She was unconscious and in shock. A massive hemorrhagic rash, spreading as we worked with her, involved her face, trunk, and extremities. A simple blood smear showed many pairs of a small round microorganism. It was clear she had an overwhelming bloodstream infection due to the meningococcus. Sulfadiazine and massive support measures were started immediately but to no avail, and she died at about 11 A.M.—nineteen hours after we had initially seen her.

In retrospect, there were several subtle clues that should have, at 4 P.M. rather than at midnight, led us to say "tilt, this might be a bacterial not a viral infection." The sudden onset of her illness, the shaking chill, the vomiting, and the immature white cells in her bloodstream were not weighted properly in the initial formulation. Separating potentially serious situations from innocent-appearing ones is not a simple process.

A second vignette illustrates a different facet of the problem. It is with considerable pride that I have recently watched my eldest daughter graduate from medical school. As a youngster and throughout her college career she has been an individual possessed of great sensivity to the needs of others. She has felt strongly about social injustice, about the needs of the downtrodden. She spent large amounts of her own free time in dealing with troubled youngsters, in tutoring those slow to learn, in working in a drug abuse center, in manning a hot line. She thought seriously of becoming a psychologist, but opted for medical school instead. I would label her a humanist by background and orientation. Yet this very same person, as a fourth year medical student, made the following statements to me after a week in the emergency room. "I hate alcoholics. If one more of them vomits on me or hits me or staggers around the emergency room cluttering up the place and interfering with my care of 'sick' patients, I think I'll kill him. I think they're disgusting. I have no patience with them. I hate to see one of them come in the door."

That would appear to have been a staggering change in my daughter's attitudes, but I think her intrinsic humanity remains. She is so anxious to acquire the scientific and technical skills with which to help people that she finds it impossible to cope as well with the inner torments of individual's so abusing themselves or with her own feelings in dealing with them. I think those deep human qualities of caring she possessed will return, but they are markedly repressed at present. There are too many other things for her to handle at this stage of her career. I had similar feelings at that point in my education, and I have seen the same reactions in many, many other young physicians.

I have borrowed the title for Part III of this book from George Bernard Shaw's play because even though Mr. Shaw held doctors in very low esteem, he realized that they did have a genuine "dilemma." I have tried with these two vignettes to capture this dilemma as I see it, to wit, how can the physician, a mere mortal, blend the qualities of compassion and caring so prized by those he treats with the rigorous and demanding science skills and knowledge that the proper application modern medicine demands? How can we select for medicine the kinds of people who can manage both well, and how can we best educate young people for this dual role? There are some delicate considerations that affect the answers to these questions. Some of the forces at play may, for instance, cause us to exclude from medicine certain people who might be fine doctors. Furthermore, many pressures tend to mold the aspiring physician in ways quite different than we might wish.

In this third part of the book, I want to approach the doctor from the inside. I have considered him at length in the preceding sections as a factor in medical care; here I wish to speak about the doctor as a person. During almost thirty years of trying to be a good doctor, coupled with my experience of educating medical students and working closely with young physicians in training during their house staff years, I have long contemplated and agonized about the process. My more recent experiences in the world outside medicine have expanded some of my perceptions regarding it. I would like to examine some of the forces that help shape the modern physician and some of the problems that young men and women face en route to becoming doctors.

I am attempting this for what I hope is a cogent reason. No matter what we wish to have as a system of medical care—how we structure it, finance it, and deploy it—it will, in the final analysis, be dependent on physicians. The physician is the only one who is equipped to go to the total pool of medical knowledge and extract from it those elements that are applicable to a given patient. So those we select for medical education and training, and the experiences—both planned and unplanned—that play upon them during their medical training and that shape them during their early years of dealing with patients, will to a great degree determine what medicine will be like. I will concentrate primarily on those experiences that engage the physician during his or her premedical education, medical school years, and initial postgraduate residency training, for those are the periods about which I know the most. I intend to examine the following areas in this section: the criteria used in selecting young men and women for medical school (Chapter 8); some of the experiences they have in their journey through medical education, particularly the dilemma of melding the science and the art of medicine—coupling technology and humanism in the delivery of patient care—and the problems that "medicalizing" certain social problems have created for today's young physicians (Chapter 9); and possible future directions in medical education (Chapter 10).

✳ *Chapter 8*

Selecting Young People
for Medical School

A problem of serious proportions, which has become increasingly intense over the last fifteen years, is the disparity between the number of openings in medical school and the number of students who apply for them. It is a simple fact that we have vastly more bright young men and women wishing to become doctors than our schools of medicine can absorb. Although we have been building medical schools at a rapid rate and have expanded the number of places for training medical students by 50 percent in the last six years, the disparity between the number who would like to go to medical school and those who can be accepted continues to widen. In 1977, the 120 medical schools in the United States enrolled over 15,000 freshman, only about one-third of the more than 45,000 individuals who had applied—most of them intelligent, well-motivated, and well-prepared young men and women.[1] The difficulty in obtaining a place in medical school is legendary—and true. This fierce competition for the available slots has of itself inevitably begun to shape the product of medical education in ways that are disquieting to many thoughtful educators and others concerned with medicine.

Why this enormous interest in medicine? In the past, students who had high interests and aptitudes in science went many other routes in addition to medicine. Some became physicists or chemists or engineers or biologists. Some opted for psychology, social work, or teaching. But during the last decade, we have seen a striking and troublesome change in the job opportunities for people with advanced graduate school training. We glutted the market with bright young Ph.D.s, and they found no room at the inn. Too many ended up driving taxis or working at jobs that made little use of their expensive training, a lesson not lost on young people or their parents. Thus, medicine has come to be one of the last professions offering independence, high status, great job satisfaction, and an excellent income. The Vietnam War also contributed to the situation. Few students were enthusiastic about entering the armed services during this period, and the draft was singularly unpopular. Graduate students in science were not deferred, but medical students were. This had quite an effect in routing science students to medicine.

This marked reduction in career options for those with professional interests has increased both the pool of medical school applicants and the tensions of those applying. "What am I going to do if I don't get into medical school?" has become an all too frequent concern. A large number of students who have been turned down by American medical schools go to other countries at great sacrifice and expense in order to obtain a medical education. Young people seem to feel, rightly or wrongly, that there are few viable alternatives.

What kinds of people apply to medical school? The motivations that prompt young people to aspire to medical careers obviously vary—but I believe less than one might think. My observations lead me to believe that most consider medicine as a career because of a genuine fondness for their fellow human beings and a deep desire to be of service to them. Medical students are characteristically very high achievers. Many people feel that it is the potential income of doctors that attracts many young people to medicine. This may have become a more important reason as other high income professions have been closed out, but I feel that income is still not a primary motivation for most. Aspiring medical students are, as a group, very curious about how things work. They are intrigued with the innards of radios, electrical circuits, machines, and the human body. They have an interest in and high aptitude for science and abstract concepts.

My own experience leads me to feel that, paradoxically, they are less scholarly and introspective than those who select such other scientific pursuits as mathematics, physics, or biochemistry, or academic careers in areas such as history, economics, or the social sciences. They are in general a motor active lot. They like to be doing things. Although there are obvious exceptions to this, they tend to be less contemplative than others who are viewed as scholars in our society.

A number of studies have attempted to characterize the kinds of people who aspire to a medical career and those that are selected for it. Dr. Daniel Funkenstein of Harvard has some interesting data suggesting that there are two types of people who move toward medicine—those with intense interest in science and research and those who are more people-oriented—and that the medical school selection process favors the scientific group.[2] In spite of this, however, most who point toward medicine have, I believe, a reasonably social and humanitarian orientation.

I am often asked why, if, as students, doctors were as people-oriented as I claim them to be, this doesn't show more. Did their experiences in becoming doctors change them or make them less sensitive to human frailties? I think the answer to this question is yes; they are changed in the process. The problem of how to prevent or minimize the loss or displacement of humanistic skills is one of the very real dilemmas of modern medicine or, more precisely, one of the problems faced by the institutions and the process that prepares young people for careers in medicine.

Medical education and the practice of medicine itself are intellectually and physically demanding. They require high skills in reading, and in comprehension, the abilities to observe accurately, in assimilating and recalling complex science constructs and being able to reason from them. Medicine also requires the ability to make decisions—often far-reaching decisions—on the basis of incomplete evidence; to tolerate worrisome ambiguities; to make reasoned judgments in emotionally distressing, often tragic situations; to work very long hours; and to maintain these abilities under circumstances of fatigue or sleep deprivation.

This is a formidable list of attributes. Those faced with the soul-searching task of selecting as candidates for medical school, young people who might possess these characteristics try to get some objective data on which to make a judgment. To do so they look carefully at how students have done in high school and college with material that was in some ways similar. How have they fared with tough science courses? Dictated in part by efforts to be reasonably objective, impartial, and fair when sifting through a vastly greater number of capable students than can be accepted, medical school admission committees place significant weight on how the student has done in biology, chemistry, physics, and higher mathematics. While considerable attention is paid to other kinds of more human but impressionistic data—how the student is viewed by his peers, how well he or she tolerates frustration, how broadly ranging his or her interest are, evidence of leadership potential, indications of coolness under stress—these kinds of attributes have proved more difficult to quantitate in our very quantifying world. The intense competition for those precious places and the increasingly litigious nature of our society has tended to make admission committees less and less adventurous and more desirous of having "hard" data on which to defend their decisions. Witness the furor over the recent Defunis and

Bakke lawsuits.[3] Both were brought against professional schools by individuals who had been refused admission who could show that their grades, scholastic aptitude tests, and the like were as good if not better than some of those admitted. Now obviously, the mere fact of high grade point averages does not the good doctor make, but the climate has pushed institutions toward more reliance on what can be measured or displayed in a ranking order to show how they made their selections in the first place. I do not believe that human skills or interest in people are deemed less important than science skills by those selecting students for medical school, but these attributes have proved much harder to get a grip on. Alas, as in many other areas of our present world, that which is more measurable may be driving out that which is more important.

THE ASPIRING PHYSICIAN'S COLLEGE CAREER

What of the medical student's college preparation—the four years of experience in an educational setting that precede medical school? How does it shape the aspiring physician? Because getting into medical school has become so distressingly competitive, most premed students concentrate very heavily on scientific courses, despite what medical school catalogues say and genuinely mean about a broad liberal education background being desirable. A liberal eduction that allows a young person to more fully know himself and his range of interests and aptitudes often goes by the board. At present, the selection system sends a certain message to young men and women who have a burning desire to be doctors: If it is medical school you aspire to, you'd be wise to take courses A through H to enhance your chances of getting a place. You should do this even if the courses are not in the areas of scholarly endeavor that currently most appeal to you. Further, whether you enjoy those courses or not, you must do very, very well in them. Straight As will be acceptable. An occasional B is perhaps tolerable. Mostly Bs will prove a disaster. Even a perfect grade point average will not guarantee you a slot in medical school, but without exemplary grades, you have no chance at all.

The result of this stressful situation is what any thoughtful person would predict. It forces young men and women who wish to be doctors to give up many areas of interest. It constricts their opportunities to explore subject material in leisurely or meandering ways that might be enlightening and shape them differently during an important formative period. They must hew sharply to scholarship in fairly restricted areas. They must perform unfailingly to shoot for a distant goal that, despite such sacrifices and purposefulness, is in no way assured.

These facts of life tend to separate this group of students quite sharply from their non-medical-school-aspiring college classmates. They have the tendency to make premedical students very single-tracked, overly competitive, and preoccupied with how they are perceived by teachers rather than with what they are acquiring or becoming. They are more interested in the outcome than the process. They focus on grades, not course content. The stresses of this life often make them resentful and cause them to feel unfulfilled. Stories about the selfishness of premedical students—their unwillingness to help fellow students—and actual destructive behavior directed at others (botching another student's chemistry experiment, discarding a classmate's notes, etc.) seem to be based in fact.

These problems, created to a great degree by the scarcity of places in medical schools, are not lost on those who are teachers of medicine and those responsible for selecting young men and women for medical careers. Medicine requires that those who practice it possess great personal integrity and honesty. It requires an ability to be a self-starter, to learn on one's own, and to have a genuine interest in the success and the welfare of others. It requires a commitment to a never-ending effort to continuously upgrade skills throughout a long professional lifetime. Those concerned with medical education and with the education that precedes it are trying to encourage the development of these characteristics, but it is proving very difficult in the situation that exists today.

※ *Chapter 9*

The Journey Through
Medical Education

For those fortunate enough to make it through the doors
of a medical school, some of the pressures are relieved.
Great efforts have gone into making the demanding experience of medical education less threatening and more collegial
than many other graduate educational endeavors. Failure rates are
low, and enormous amounts of faculty time and energy are devoted
to trying to help each student who enters successfully through to his
or her medical degree. But there are dilemmas, nevertheless. In arriving at medical school, students are inclined to feel: Okay, I wanted
to work with people and to learn how to cope with their problems.
I have spent four very demanding years of college setting aside these
interests and successfully completing many courses that seemed far
removed from my goals. I am now ready to learn about human function and illness and how to cure disease.

Once again, the student is asked to postpone these kinds of
gratifications. The message he receives back is: We understand that,
but first we will ask you to spend two years learning the language
and the scientific underpinnings of medicine. You will be required to
have a thorough knowledge of anatomy, histology, biochemistry,
microbiology, immunology, physiology, pharmacology, and the like
before we will let you have the privilege of interacting with your
potential patients. Many of these courses, indeed most of them, will
be taught by splendid scientists who have and are making the kinds
of basic scientific contributions on which modern medicine is based.
But you should understand that they often march to a different
drummer than you do. Their interests are quite appropriately focused on cells and molecules and biochemical and enzymatic
processes, not on intact human beings. Furthermore, some rather

115

resent the time and energy they must spend in trying to impart their subject matter and their excitement about their science to you who have your eye on a quite different target. Thus, because they are human, they may occasionally appear to take their frustration out on you. But make no mistake, you must master these subjects to their satisfaction. To do so you will have to work very hard—indeed, much harder than you've ever worked before. You will be surrounded by other students, all of whom will seem even brighter than you are. When you have jumped these hurdles, we will then introduce you to some of the excitements and mysteries of clinical medicine."

Obviously, this is overstating the case. Most schools are now introducing students to patients and beginning to let them acquire skills in interviewing and working with sick and troubled people early on, while they are simultaneously acquiring these basic science tools. I would wager, however, that most medical students today would agree with my characterization of how the first two years of medical school appear to them.

Medical school is a demanding and often quite isolated life. The rigor of the experience, the workload that forces young men and women to spend evenings and sunny Saturdays and Sundays in the anatomy laboratory or poring over books or working with very sick patients separates them quite sharply from their college classmates who have gone other directions.

Coming quite abruptly and intensely into contact with death and the process of dying—particularly with the deaths of people one's own age or younger—also tends to make the medical student a different person. In American society at large, most people face death in its tangible forms very infrequently. With the exception of an occasional aged grandparent, seldom do young people observe a person undergoing this ultimate struggle or have to cope with its effects on husbands, wives, parents, or others that it touches. Some rapid personal adjustments and adaptations are required for the medical student to manage this continuing reality without being overwhelmed by it. It sometimes is hard to listen to what appear to be trivial concerns of healthy people working in other pursuits when one has just come from total immersion in some stark tragedy in the hospital. I can vividly remember my own feelings of separateness from college friends when we got together. They discussed buying homes or having families or canoeing on weekends or going to the theater or museums. I lived in a dormitory, hit the books, and tried to help sick patients, many of whom ended up dead. Because it is painful for young people to watch other kinds of life passing by, the medical student tends to withdraw from such outside contacts. It is also the stark difference in the medical students' world from that of others that causes this withdrawal. To a degree, it resembles the phenomenom of those who have undergone painful wartime experiences and are unwilling to talk about them. In part, it is the unwillingness to relive the horror. In part, however, it also stems from a resignation to the fact that people outside the medical world simply cannot comprehend what those inside are talking about. Therefore, one's contacts in medical school become largely one's fellow medical students, who have similar aspirations, similar anxieties, similar feelings of deprivation, and similar struggles with some of life's most unpleasant realities.

The selection of a medical career requires that one give up, at least for a time, many interests or skills that made the medical student the kind of person he was prior to entry. Artistic interests and participation in sports and the outdoor life must all be sharply curtailed or set aside. Dr. Rene Dubos once told me, "Each career decision one makes means that an individual murders one kind of self that one might have been." He developed this thought beautifully in his biography of Louis Pasteur:

> There is drama in the thought that every time we make a choice, turn right instead of left, pronounce one word instead of another, we favor one of our potential beings at the expense of all the rest of our personality—nay, we likely starve and smother to death something of us that could have continued to grow. Every decision is like a murder, and our march forward is over the stillborn bodies of all of our possible selves that will never be. But such is the penalty of a productive life.[1]

This is, I believe, particularly true in the case of those opting for a career in medicine. Although some interests or hobbies or skills can be reacquired at a later date, it is nevertheless painful to have to give them up, and some are never recaptured.

COUPLING SCIENCE AND HUMANISM IN MEDICINE

One of the difficulties experienced by aspiring young physicians (and established ones, too) is the problem of how to reconcile their concern for the welfare of people with the scientific and technologic requirements of medicine. This is a dilemma of this century—as a matter of fact, of the last thirty years. It simply did not exist before. The doctor of yore—the familiar television doc of "Gunsmoke" days—had little other than his compassion, his knowledge of the patient and his family, and his understanding of

the natural history of disease with which to work. Fond remin-
iscences to the contrary, there was precious little that he could really
do except to control bleeding, relieve pain, treat malaria, set frac-
tured bones, do simple kinds of surgery, or aid in difficult deliveries.
But starting in the 1920s with the discovery of insulin and moving at
a progressively rapid rate since then, the march of science-based
medicine began to change all of this. During the last thirty years,
we have amassed an impressive amount of knowledge about the
human organism and about disease and how to manipulate it. We
now have many tools that allow precise diagnosis and multiple agents
and therapies that can either cure disease or drastically modify its
effects. Dr. Grey Dimond, a distinguished physician who graduated
in the early 1940s, recently made the point that practically nothing
that he was taught in medical school in the 1940s was useful to him
or even necessarily accurate in 1976. (I believe this overstates the
case. As a matter of fact, I have been amazed throughout my professional life at how sound and current were basic skills I learned
thirty years ago.) He then listed the medical aids for patient care that
were unknown or largely unavailable to him when he entered medicine. The list included antibiotics; blood transfusions; poliomyelitis
vaccine; specific medical therapies for tuberculosis, hormonal and
enzyme insufficiencies; cardiac catherization, angiography, cardiac
monitoring, defibrillation, cardiac pace makers, cardiopulmonary
bypasses, heart and great vessel surgery, and heart valve replacements; renal transplants and renal dialysis; limb replacements, organ
transplants, joint replacements; deafness surgery; lasar, radar, sonar,
and fiberoptics; nuclear medicine; concept of immune mechanisms;
and cancer chemotherapy.[2] While I might argue some specific items,
this is a staggering list! The number of technical and scientific
skills and understanding that must be assimilated by the physician
of today is immense and ever changing. Young physicians are vividly
aware of this and are struggling to acquire this knowledge. Knowing
that there are effective tools and agents available for modifying or
curing disease, they are understandably preoccupied with not missing
potentially correctable conditions in their patients.

One of the compelling forces that motivates good physicians is
fear—fear that one will miss an important clue, overlook a serious
problem, or treat as trivial something that turns out not to be. Most
physicians are constructively scared most of their professional lives.
The ring of the telephone evokes a conditioned reaction: Will I be
able to cope with the problem that is about to present itself? Is this
patient with a headache reacting to the tensions of his life or does he
have a malignant hypertension, meningitis, or a brain tumor? Is the

deterioration in the behavior pattern of this young woman due to a broken marriage, a parathyroid adenoma, declining kidney function, adrenal or thyroid insufficiency, or the medications she is taking? Considerable knowledge and sometimes subjecting the patient to a number of expensive and/or uncomfortable procedures are required to make these kinds of differential diagnoses. The aspiring young physician must know the different diagnostic possibilities and how to weigh them. He must also be familiar with the various tests and procedures available to enhance his diagnostic skills and the alternative possibilities for treatment. The good physician can muster a broader array of possibilities and weigh them more accurately than a poor one. Consequently, during his training, signs of *omission*—possibilities that the young physician has failed to consider in arriving at a diagnosis for a particular patient—are frequently brought to his attention. He is continually working to expand his data base—to leave nothing out. (There is a familiar gag in medical circles when referring to a negative finding on some key diagnostic test: "It may not have helped her, but it sure did me a lot of good.") Because of this emphasis on the thoroughness, sins of *commission*— that is, including possibilities that are not germane—are not similarly emphasized in medical schools. This leads to some of the problems of overdiagnosis and overuse of technology that are being criticized today. I well remember that during my own medical training, my colleagues and I felt very badly when we missed the murmur of mitral stenosis in patients who had possible rheumatic heart disease. This was considered a sin despite the fact that at that time there was precious little we could do to change the course of events that often dramatically shortened the lives of people with this kind of heart valve damage. Few of us, however, were criticized for hearing a murmur of mitral stenosis when it was not actually present, despite the gloomy prognosis it implied. Some years later, however, when I was running a cardiac clinic for young pregnant women, I saw a significant number of young women who had been made psychological cripples by overdiagnosis of mitral stenosis when it was not present. Sins of commission can be as destructive as those of omission.

A recent paper by a thoughtful physician has made this point in a somewhat different way. Dr. Clifton Meador of Vanderbilt University has just reported careful observations on seventy-eight patients with significant and troubling symptoms whom he followed for two to four years without being able to find any diagnosable disease or definable physiologic dysfunction. It was his belief that these patients had developed their problems as a reaction to stressful life situations. The possible relationship of their symptoms to stress was acknowledged by about one-third of those patients. These patients he was able to help, and they improved. In another third of the group, this insight came with more difficulty, and he was less successful. The final third of the patients, however, denied being under any stress and continued to insist that some disease was present; with them, little or no progress was made. More germane to the point I have been making about overdiagnosis, physicians had agreed with this last group of patients with distressing frequency and in essence had "given them a disease" on which to ruminate. The twenty-nine patients who denied that stress might play any role in making them unwell had had their symptoms an average of almost eight years and collectively carried twenty-one "medical" diagnoses. Among them, they had undergone ninety-six operative procedures. Twenty-one were taking potent drugs.[3] Clearly, this is not good medicine, but it does seem indicative of the physician's compulsion to put a "label" on patients and to do something for or to them.

These kinds of problems have made me feel that we have the educational situation turned around. Overdiagnosis or overuse of diagnostic tests or technologies or drugs—sins of commission—should be viewed as errors as serious as, or even more serious than, the failure to consider all the possibilities.[4]

Be that as it may, the process of medical education stress acquisition of broad knowledge of all the diagnostic possibilities, the tests that can be brought to bear to rule them in or out, and the interventions that can be made. Acquiring this knowledge and the skills permitting its use requires enormous effort. Human caring skills are not similarly emphasized and sometimes tend to get lost or shunted aside in the process. Thus, I believe it is commonplace for young physicians to feel, "I know my own humanity, I grew up with it, and it is an important part of me. It is why I embarked on this career. But at the moment, I must set it aside. I must learn the science and the technology of medicine and must have it well in hand to avoid having people die or be harmed by disease I have missed."

Almost ninety years ago, at the opening of the Johns Hopkins Hospital in Baltimore in 1889, John Shaw Billings stated, "Affection and zeal may do much, but they cannot take the place of knowledge."[5] This ethic prevails to an even greater degree in medicine today. We live in an era of great expectations about technology and how it can help us. Clearly, much science-based technology can be applied by medicine for the great benefit of man, but it is a two-edged sword. Much of our technology of itself carries some hazards. Its use is frightening to those who receive it. It is often painful and upsetting to undergo. It is expensive. Today's physicians are therefore in a quandary. To take appropriate care of their patients—to proceed with what they view as technologically and scientifically sound management of their patients—they must often be advocates of procedures that hurt, scare, and sometimes alienate. The physician-patient relationship is often damaged in the process. The application of these new technologies poses the hazard of setting the physician and the patient apart.

Consider the hypothetical case of a young woman admitted with a high fever and profound trouble in breathing. A young physician wants to be human and caring, but he also wants to be sure not to miss the proper diagnosis. He wants to understand and cope with the worries this young woman has about herself, her separation from her family, and her being in the hospital with all kinds of frightening pieces of apparatus about. On the other hand, he feels obligated to determine whether she has a serious bacterial pneumonia or has thrown multiple blood clots to her lungs. He recognizes that he can treat either of these conditions satisfactorily, but the treatments are quite different, and he must know which problem is present. To make this differentiation, he may be forced to do a number of unpleasant and frightening things to her. He has to send her to the x-ray room to obtain a series of x-rays. This itself is often a grueling experience. He may have to puncture one of her femoral blood vessels, insert a catheter and advance it up to her heart and then inject dye into her blood stream to determine whether blood vessels in her lung are blocked off—an unpleasant and expensive procedure. He may have to put a needle into her neck and puncture her trachea to get cultures to determine whether a bacterial pneumonia is present. He may have to help her breathe using a complicated piece of equipment to deliver oxygen that is life saving, but the machine and mask are frightening. In his judgment (and, if well managed, in hers), it is worth the price. If he can diagnose the illness properly and manage it correctly, she will be totally well in a surprisingly short period of time. If he is wrong, she may not survive. The dilemma is very real and very common.

Paradoxically, new technologies have also made the care and management of patients with certain life-threatening illnesses much more demanding and time consuming for young physicians during their residency years. Consider the management of an individual with a massive myocardial infarction—a serious and potentially fatal heart attack—as I dealt with it in 1948 when I was a resident in contrast to the care such a patient might receive in 1977. In 1948, if the damage to the heart muscle was sufficiently severe to create profound heart failure or to change the heart rhythm so that it failed to pump sufficient blood, the patient generally died quite promptly. I did what I could, generally by myself with the assistance of a nurse, but my tools were limited, and the issue was generally decided in a matter of several hours. A patient with a similar episode who is admitted today can be aided by a remarkable series of measures and devices that can support the failing heart, even do its pumping for it. Drugs can prevent fatal rhythm abnormalities, or abnormalities can be halted and normal rhythm restored, even if the heart stops. A young resident nowadays may spend eithteen to twenty-four continuous hours with this patient, assisted by a large cadre of skilled nurses, technicians, and machines in applying these marvelous technical tools. An individual who would have died in 1948 may be restored to full activity in 1977, but the costs in time, people, and machines of taking care of him has been markedly increased.

THE MEDICALIZATION OF MANY SOCIAL PROBLEMS

In a previous chapter, I described the dilemma that the "Medicalization" of many problems previously not considered in the purview of medicine has created for academic medical centers. The passing parade of troubled people who seek help for these problems from those working in busy teaching hospitals also tends to shape the character and attitudes of the young physician in training in ways not always positive.

As I have already indicated, those who become medical students are characteristically high achievers. Indeed, they must have been so quite consistently to be admitted to medical school. They have been unerringly "successful," as gauged by the yardstick of our society. They are selected as medical students in part because they have conformed to the dictates of our educational and social systems. They have never failed. They are some of the most successful "copers" of our world.

But in the academic medical center's teaching hospital—in its clinics, its emergency room, and on its wards—they are faced daily with the problems of many people who are unable to make satisfactory adjustments to our world. They see men and women who neglect and beat their children. They daily encounter individuals who overuse alcohol to such a degree that they are destroying their bodies and their brains. They see young people with the dreadful diseases produced by intravenous injections of mind-altering drugs. In such situations, where the physician in training is often tired and lacks the necessary tools to manage these problems, he or she is frequently depressed, often appalled, and sometimes angry about the human misery that marches before his eyes. Unused to failure in themselves, these young doctors have difficulty understanding or identifying with the tragic human failures they see. Indeed, their own humanity often makes managing these patients even more difficult for them. In an effort to deal with these very tense situations, they frequently repress their own emotions and caring tendencies. The feeling is often, "I will deal with the massive gastroentestinal bleeding, I will deal with this impending liver coma in this alcoholic derelict but I will not at present try to understand or cope with the human being who has done these awful things to himself. I will think about the deranged physiology of liver coma and take steps to correct it, I will replace the blood and fluids that are lost, but I will not consider this individual as human. That is too difficult for me to contemplate."

These experiences, and the science orientation of most of the faculty with whom medical students come in contact, tends to make the young doctors more detached, apparently more impersonal and analytic, than they were at the outset of medical education. Studies by Dr. Daniel Funkenstein have documented that such a shift occurs. Fifty percent of the students surveyed upon entry into Harvard Medical School wished to become "clinicians" and 25 percent "scientists." By graduation, the percentages were almost reversed—fewer than 30 percent were pointing toward careers as clinicians while almost 40 percent wished to have careers in medical science. These figures become more disquieting as one examines the characteristics of these two types of students as described by Funkenstein:

The Student-Scientist. These students' primary value is to be a scientist, and secondarily to be of service through research. The treatment of patients is in a tertiary position and is viewed as a science. This is well illustrated by their response when asked to check a number of activities which they consider important in their careers as physicians. Almost none of the students checked "working with people"; almost all checked "to be creative and original in science." Introspection was a very minor value.

These students are similar in many of their characteristics to graduate students in the basic sciences. They have high quantitative aptitudes and have carried the study of science far forward in college. At the time of admission to medical school, they are still debating whether they should work toward a Ph.D. or an M.D. degree.

The Student-Clinician. These students are primarily interested in working with people, in service to people by directly helping them, and in applying pragmatically the basic sciences which are applicable to the diagnosis and treatment of patients. Introspection occupies a low place in their value hierarchy. In college they majored in extracurricular activities, usually occupying leadership positions on campus. Their aptitude scores are not as high as those of the other two groups of students. An increasing number of these future physicians are interested in dealing directly with social problems, and exercising leadership in delivering medical care.[6]

Another study on medical students, conducted by Harrison Gough and Wallace Hall, is also less than reassuring about the characteristics that students both lose and acquire in transit through medical school. For those viewed as most successful as medical students, their colleagues employed such adjectives as "silent," "insightful," "realistic," "logical," and "foresighted." Students rated least successful were characterized as "unselfish," "sentimental," and "softhearted."[7] Further work by Gough also suggests that students ranking as most creative do not necessarily fare better than average in medical school.[8]

It is not all bad. The same study also demonstrated that students respond to the stresses of medical school by developing enhanced problem-solving capabilities and firmer resolve to follow through on tough tasks.

We are trying to walk a tricky tight rope here.

What I believe we are seeking to develop in the fully formed doctor is a person who not only develops and maintains high science skills but also retains and is fully comfortable with his or her human qualities of caring and compassion. These qualities should also be regarded as skills—potent therapeutic tools—to be developed and used.

The term "detached compassion" is sometimes used to describe the kind of relationship a physician should have with his patients. By this is meant that without any great display of emotion, the physician can demonstrate by his actions and demeanor that he recognizes, understands, and will seek to allay his patients' anxiety, depression, or grief as well as their physical symptoms. However, "detached compassion" does not quite capture all the qualities that I feel the fully formed physician should have. He must also learn to not pass judgment on his fellow man and to empathize with those requiring care. Indeed, there are times when compassion need not be so detached. A truly secure physician can sometimes put his arms around a patient, or hold his or her hand, or even shed a few tears with a bereaved wife or son or mother. It is a sensitive and delicate role to play, and how to do it best remains a doctor's dilemma.

Chapter 10

Future Directions
for Medical Education

In describing some of the forces that help shape the aspiring physicians, I have primarily emphasized those that can interfere with or distort his or her development as the "compleat physician." It is worth emphasizing, however, that despite these pressures, most young men and women who move through these experiences to become doctors come out quite well formed. Bright students have a remarkable capacity to learn from what is good and to discard what is bad in the educational environment, and much that is good and inspiring is encountered in the process of being educated for a medical career.

There is the realization that one is acquiring knowledge and skills that will permit one to help fellow humans through some of life's travails. This is heady wine. That it requires enormous effort, the assimilation of a large body of factual information, and dogged persistance merely enhances the worth of attaining this knowledge and skill.

Also, as is so often the case, such an intense experience often brings out the best as well as the worst in people, and the medical student is continually exposed to some remarkable illustrations of inspired human performance. The medical student works very closely with many others of varying experience, all dedicated to achieving similar objectives. Learning by working with others toward a common goal is a vivid experience that generally creates real personal growth and lasting insights. There are many impressive "models" to observe among one's fellow students, residents, and faculty. These contacts tend to enrich and expand the goals to which young physicians aspire or their concept of what they themselves might become.

Clinical education as it has evolved has some considerable educational strengths. Medical school faculty live in glass houses. Although students complain that lectures are overused, those who teach clinical medicine spend much time in unstructured small group sessions. They must practice what they profess, on ward rounds, in the clinics, and in interactions with students and house staff who share in the care of their patients. Thus, the aspiring physician daily sees his mentors in the stressful give and take of working with sick people. The student can see how the professor actually behaves in real life situations working on real problems—something quite rare in other educational settings. There is considerable democracy in medical education. In the best of clinical settings, it is the nature of the evidence, not your age or rank, that takes precedence in patient care. This creates a certain collegiality and free exchange of information that is not found in most educational experiences.

But these important strengths in medical education do not mean that those in the business can ignore the forces that I have cited that tend to make the doctor less than he or she might become. We select for medical school high achievers who, by virtue of the fact that they function so well under pressure, are at risk of being less sensitive to the needs of those less able to cope with the pressures of modern society. We put them through an intense science-oriented education that isolates them from others and runs the risk of making them more detached, less emotionally involved with others, and more cynical. We do not adequately reward aspiring physicians for humanitarian skills. How might we improve the process?

Virtually all those in educational circles who deal either with premedical education or with the selection of young men and women for medicine are now deeply concerned about the unusual pressures that have been created by the fierce competition for places in medical school and what those pressures are doing to potential doctors. This country has been building new medical schools at a rapid rate for over a decade, and there are yet more on the drawing board. Indeed, there is much to suggest that we are well on our way to the overproduction of physicians at what will represent great cost to the nation.[1] But the numbers of students wishing entry to medical school has kept pace with or exceeded the increase in the number of openings and will probably continue to do so. Competition for admission has not and probably will not be eliminated by simply expanding medical school places. Consequently, other ways of reducing the stresses caused by this competition need exploration.

EARLY ADMISSION FOR SOME STUDENTS

One approach would be to settle the entry question well before the fact. Certain institutions are conducting experiments in early acceptance or early entry into medical school. Some are awarding places in medical school to promising students well before the actual time of entry, believing that assurance of a place in medical school will relieve some of the anxieties and permit students to broaden and gain more from their college experience. Other schools are letting students begin medical school with less preparation. For many years, Johns Hopkins permitted some students to enter medical school after two or three years of college, taking a transitional year in which medically oriented courses and liberal arts college courses were combined to ease the assimilation into medicine. The track record of these students compared favorably with those going the traditional route. Certain institutions, notably the University of Missouri at Kansas City and the City College of New York, are now accepting promising premedical students at a younger age. Each has a six year curriculum, with entry into a medical track directly from high school. Each of these institutions has found ways of decompressing the medical curriculum and interdigitating it with a broader exposure to English, history, the arts, and the social sciences, which makes for better-educated men and women.

These experiments look interesting and promising to me. They do eliminate some of the cutthroat pressure of premedical education for those who have made an early career choice. They do not, however, solve the problem for a number of people who make much later decisions to move toward medicine. We need these more mature students as well. Individuals who have sampled alternative lifestyles or worked in the Peace Corps or Vista or the Urban League are not much in evidence in medical schools. We need ways of offering some medical school slots to such people who have differing perceptions of our world.

TEACH MORE HUMAN BIOLOGY IN COLLEGE

Another way to tackle the entry pressure problem would be to move a considerable amount of what is now taught during the first two years of medical school back to college campuses. I have long believed that introducing young people to the wonders of human biology much earlier on in their careers makes great sense. Educated people should know more about how they are put together and function, and it would enrich and strengthen college offerings in the process.[2] Further, I believe this move might help expand the thinking of young people about the career possibilities in other biological and social service professions in addition to medicine. The fields of anthropology, social work, psychology, biochemistry, pharmacy, health care administration, and public health might be better served if college age students knew more of what they had to offer.

Modern biomedical science has now progressed to a place where many fundamental insights of broad interest to educated people can be taught from human examples. It has always seemed strange to me that we expect "educated" people to have a comfortable acquaintance with English, mathematics, history, literature, and so forth without similarly expecting them to know considerable amounts about human biology and psychology. Young people entering college are deeply interested in what makes them function as they do—both physically and emotionally. To take advantage of these interests and concerns in designing educational offerings seems to me eminently sensible. Why not teach the science of genetics—which includes considerable amounts of mathematics, logic, probability theory, and the like—with human examples rather than the fruit fly? The age when people are especially concerned about why they behave as they do—why they feel shy or angry or depressed or uncertain—seems a wonderful time to teach introductory human psychology and sociology—and why not from human examples rather than from studies on rats or lower animals? We have certainly demonstrated that young people can comfortably assimilate much more complicated material in grade school and high school than previously supposed. Children now acquire skills in mathematics by the time they enter high school that are well beyond those I learned in college. It seems probable that this could be the case with other rigorous disciplines.

Introducing a biomedical approach to the science and social science curricula of colleges would permit medical school faculties to deal with their complex subject matter at a higher level and could help to make medical school education more flexible. Some colleges are now moving in this direction. They need vigorous encouragement by those in medicine.

BROADEN SELECTION CRITERIA

Many medical schools recognize that their current ways of selecting students are not satisfactory—that they are measuring and quantitating skills and attributes that are only moderately well correlated with the attributes that are most important in fully formed doctors. This became very apparent as medical schools began concerted efforts to enroll more minority students. The deficiencies in current testing procedures—their cultural, educational, and attitudinal biases—became glaringly evident. It became obvious that we were selecting as candidates for medical school a fairly monochromatic group of students who looked, thought, and acted similarly and who had very similar educational and experiential backgrounds. This does not serve medicine well or the variegated public that medicine in turn serves. We need physicians with backgrounds in Spanish-speaking, black, or American Indian culture. A number of efforts are now under way to broaden and improve the instruments used in the identification and selection of capable individuals from these backgrounds.

There is evidence that advancing knowledge in behavioral science may allow better assessment of more subtle human attributes than mere intellectual horsepower. Twelve medical schools are currently working with experts from the National Board of Medical Examiners and the Educational Testing Service to try to formulate tests structured to yield information about characteristics and aptitudes that correlate well with success in clinical medicine and that are not captured by current ways of evaluating students or by simple interviews. The Association of American Medical Colleges has just extensively revised the Medical College Aptitude Test in an effort to remove cultural or background biases. I hope these efforts will broaden the spectrum of people in our medical schools.

INTRODUCE HUMAN INTERACTION SKILLS
EARLIER IN THE CURRICULUM

At the same time, many medical schools are beginning to introduce students to patients early in their medical education. Here they are making use of the knowledge from the behavioral sciences to develop interviewing skills and a more sophisticated understanding of the power of the doctor-patient relationship and to make students better aware of their own attitudes and how they affect their care of others. The basic sciences are increasingly interdigitated with these learnings. Because many of the basic sciences germane to medicine assume increasing importance in the student's mind only after he is faced with some of the clinical problems that he encounters in the third and fourth years, a number of schools are reintroducing basic science courses during the latter half of medical school. Most schools have dramatically shortened certain didactic courses like gross anatomy and have expanded teaching in areas where there is an interface between basic science and clinical practice, such as clinical pharmacology.

Some institutions are also attempting to make the medical school more conscious of the "humanness" of all of us. The experiments now being conducted at McMasters University in Canada look interesting in this regard and deserve careful study. The McMasters Medical School was founded only eight years ago, and its first dean was a strong believer in innovative education. He chose the core faculty both for their medical competence and for their willingness to let students be more responsible for their own education. Faculty attitudes as well as their professional skills and knowledge were deemed important.

At McMasters, a new student is assigned to a small group of five, with a tutor. This group functions as a learning group for about ten weeks. In phases of approximately ten weeks each, the student is a member of successive groups, always kept to five in number. From the first day, students begin working on the medical problems with which they will eventually be faced. They start with case material: Here is a patient with such and such symptoms. What are you going to do? What do you want to know in order to decide what to do? The group discussion is at all times open to feelings as well as to ideas. Thus, students may well feel totally inadequate in dealing with their first "case," competitive with others, insecure in a new situation. Such feelings are as acceptable as the many ideas about how to gain the information needed for proper diagnosis and management. The group soon breaks up to go about obtaining the knowledge they need. All the resources of the medical school are open to them for their learning. Then they gather to pool their learnings and make diagnoses and treatment decisions. Finally, they are told the actual diagnosis, what was actually done, and the outcome.

As they progress through studying past medical records, working with "simulated patients," and dealing with real patients who are being cared for by other physicians, they are allowed to carry more and more responsibility themselves for actual patients. The medical curriculum, as it is usually understood, does not exist. There is no traditional course in anatomy, for example. The student is encouraged to learn what he or she wants and needs to find out in order to deal with a problem that is real to him. It is truly self-directed learning, very complex in its interspecialty and interdisciplinary searchings.

A number of things have been learned in this process. It is found that the tutor need not be an expert in the problem under consideration. Sometimes, in fact, the nonexpert tutor is more effective than the expert. (When the medical problem falls within the tutor's special competence, he or she is more likely to forget the facilitative role and to become an authority, a lecturer.)

Another insight is that there is a recurrent tension in the group between the desire to learn the necessary cognitive facts and the desire to deal with the personal feelings and needs of the members. Learning in this fashion does not go smoothly, but seems to pass back and forth from the cognitive to the affective. As in all medical education, the desire to know the facts and to acquire the science skills is very strong. Yet the personal aspect is not forgotten, and a student's peers and faculty are open to his personal concerns.

So far, the outcome of this most unorthodox approach looks promising. Although McMaster's is a three year medical school, its students' record in the Canadian licensing examination compares well with that of the other schools. For example, for the past four years, they have consistently performed above the Canadian national average in medicine, psychiatry, and public health, about average in pediatrics, and slightly below average in obstetrics and surgery. No great emphasis is placed on this record by the faculty, because this examination measures only medical knowledge and not the many other objectives that the school has chosen. The morale of their graduates is high, and they seem to find that their medical education encourages them to place a higher value on their human qualities than do students in other schools.[3]

Efforts to help faculty be more aware of how their feelings and attitudes and interactions with others influence their effectiveness as physicians or teachers are also expanding in this country. Group workshops entitled Human Dimensions in Medical Education that have been conducted under the auspices of the Center for the Study of the Person in La Jolla, California, have involved over 500 senior faculty from more than fifty schools. One developing medical school, East Virginia, in Norfolk, is also making use of a group of the center's staff to design their curriculum and faculty-student relationships in new and more collegial ways. A program conducted by the Association of American Medical Colleges has also been directed at improving the human and managerial skills of those who teach medicine. Thus, a number of medical schools are directing considerable attention to how they can better meld science and humanism in medicine.

Some years ago, I wrote an article entitled "The Doctor Himself Must Become the Treatment," in which I indicated that physicians often fail to recognize how important understanding and support can be in their therapeutic armamentarium.[4] Some of it I borrowed from Dr. Jeremiah Barondess as well.[5] I said:

> ...a disease is a biologic event of a pathologic sort. It is something that happens to a cell, or to a molecule, or to an organ, or even to an entire organism. Disease is a *biologic* process that can be understood in scientific and objective terms.
>
> An illness, on the other hand, is a *human* event. It is a grouping of discomforts, dysfunctions, anxieties, changes in feeling state and the ability to function which occurs in a *person*....Illness is...an event in the course of human life. It is often of great importance (to) the individual who is experiencing it. It is embedded in the trappings of concerns, responsibilities, hopes, and fears of that special and unique and particular person. Thus, an illness is ultimately to be understood not in scientific, but in human terms.
>
> *Both* disease and illness are the proper purview of medicine. Physicians can cure but a few *diseases*....But the fully formed physician should be prepared and willing to treat most if not all *illnesses*, and somewhere along the line in our scientific transformation this obvious absolutely basic and fundamental mission of the physician seems to have been mislaid.

I quote that statement because I like it—but I now believe it an error to separate "science" and "humanism" in such a polar way. A number of psychiatrists and psychologists have pointed out that humanism can also be scientific. A considerable body of scientific data about human feelings, behavior, and interactions is developing that can be taught to and assimilated by physicians. These skills, formerly acquired by trial and error, can make doctors considerably more comfortable and more adept at coping with problems not subject to technologic manipulation. It seems likely that medicine has for too long stubbornly clung to the view that the study of disease is a "science" while the care of the patient is an "art."

Dr. George Engel of Rochester has written persuasively on this subject.[6] He points out that in the care of the patient, understanding him, knowing what is going on within his brain and his psyche as well as his physiology, is as much a matter for science as the study of disease. Ways of dealing with feeling states, attitudes, or abberant behavior can now be predicated on reliable data and are amenable to validation and scientific study in no way different from other facets of medicine. If we can teach humanism more scientifically and put more understanding of its uses in the hands of those who practice medicine, I think we will better address the problems that trouble people most about their physicians. Gaps in communication and a failure to develop a healthy, therapeutic doctor-patient relationship seem the basis for many of the dissatisfactions that patients have with their doctors and are responsible for many if not most of the malpractice suits being filed today. Such humanistic skills might also permit young physicians to cope better with their personal anxieties and attitudes and allow medical people to deal more comfortably with the "medicalized" social problems that increasingly confront them.

But as I indicated in Chapter 5, given the current state of knowledge, many of the social problems now shunted to medicine cannot be solved by physicians working in isolation. Some would go so far as to argue that the physician, given his background, attitudes, and training, may be the least able to work effectively with these illnesses, not least of all because he is perceived as an authority figure. Such advocates feel that others with different kinds of training or experiences would be more successful. While this may in part be the case (indeed, ex-drug addicts and ex-alcoholics have been more effective as therapists than doctors in a number of settings), it isn't necessarily so. Granted, the physician who is rigid and insecure does not do well in these settings. However a really good doctor can often operate effectively in these areas. If someone is to help others, he or she must radiate the ability to help. Such skills characterize the best physicians, and I think they will remain involved. But, at the very least, physicians must form new alliances with others to better manage such illnesses. A number of institutions are creating "teams" composed of physicians and those trained in nursing, social service, psychology, the ministry, education, and the like to cope better with these transmedical problems. The growth of new groups and institutions devoting their attention to what has been termed "humanistic" or "holistic" medicine is clearly an effort to take a broader view of healing.[7] We should critically evaluate the results achieved by these groups; but finding new ways to approach human problems deserves encouragement.

The physician will remain key to the delivery of medical care. Many of my suggestions for reducing some of the less desirable pressures on him during his formative period are already being tested. Institutions are studying ways to broaden the student mix entering medicine. A number are changing the sequence and scope of subject matter offered to students in medical schools and are giving more attention to the development of humanistic skills, though this goes slowly. Certain institutions and physicians are forming alliances with other disciplines to better manage problems not subject to present medical technology and are widening the perceptions of what constitutes healing.

The physician will remain a fallible human being, subject to the same frailties that plague us all. Ways that will permit him to cope better with the tasks we have assigned him should make him a yet more effective force in our complex modern world.

References

PART I – INTRODUCTION

1. "What Do People Pray About? Health is Concern of Most According to FCL Analysis," *Pawling News Chronical* (Pawling, New York), May 11, 1977, p. 1

2. David E. Rogers and Robert J. Blendon, "The Changing American Health Scene: Sometimes Things Get Better," *Journal of the American Medical Association*, 237, no. 16 (April 18, 1977): 1710-13.

3. David E. Rogers, "One Foundation's Aspirations," The President's Statement, *The Robert Wood Johnson Foundation Annual Report 1972.* (Philadelphia: Wm. F. Fell Company, 1972).

CHAPTER 1

1. Quoted in Robert H. Ebert, "The Medical School," in *Life and Death and Medicine*, edited by the staff of *Scientific American* (San Francisco: W.H. Freeman and Company, 1973), p. 103.

2. Ibid.

3. Abraham Flexner, *Medical Education in the United States and Canada: A Report to the Carnegie Foundation for the Advancement of Teaching* (New York: The Carnegie Foundation, 1910).

4. Quoted in John H. Knowles, "The Hospital," in *Life and Death and Medicine*, edited by the staff of *Scientific American* (San Francisco: W.H. Freeman and Company, 1973), p. 92.

5. David E. Rogers, "Setting of Priorities for Health Care Delivery," *Clinical Research* 25, no. 4 (October 1977): Table 8.

6. Julius B. Richmond, "The Needs of Children," *Daedalus* 106, no. 1 (Winter 1977): 247-49.

7. *Sourcebook of Health Insurance Data 1976-77* (New York: Health Insurance Institute, 1977).

CHAPTER 2

1. National Center for Health Statistics, *Vital and Health Statistics, Current Estimates from Health Interview. Survey, United States, July 1966–June 1967*, Series 10, no. 43 (January 1968), Tables 16 and 17.

2. David E. Rogers and Robert J. Blendon, "The Changing American Health Scene: Sometimes Things Get Better," *Journal of the American Medical Association* 237, no. 16 (April 18, 1977): Table 1.

3. Figures apply to the civilian and noninstitutionalized populations only. National Center for Health Statistics, *Vital and Health Statistics*, series 10, no. 119 (November 1977), Tables 20 and 21.

4. Rogers and Blendon, pp. 1710–13.

5. Ibid., pp. 1711–12.

6. Association of American Medical Colleges, *Medical School Admission Requirements*, 1967 and 1977 eds. (Washington, D.C., January 1968, January 1978).

7. National Center for Health Statistics, *Health Resources Statistics*, 1975 (U.S. National Center for Statistics, Rockville, Md., 1976).

8. American Dental Association, *Dental Education Annual Report* (Chicago: National Dental Association, 1967 and 1977).

9. American Medical Association, *Allied Health Education Fact Sheet* (Chicago: American Medical Associaion, March 1977).

10. National Center for Health Statistics, *Infant Mortality Rates: Socioeconomic Factors*, series 22, no. 14, DHEW Publication No. (JSM) 72-1045 (Washington, D.C.: Government Printing Office, 1972).

11. D.S. Kessner, *Infant Death: An Analysis of Maternal Risk and Health Care* (Washington, D.C.: Institute of Medicine/National Academy of Sciences, 1973).

12. G. Issacs, "A Universal Model for Health Care, or the Dilemma of a Primary Health Care Agency in a Medically Oriented Society" (Paper read at the International Health Conference Program, Arlington, Virginia, October 1975.

13. E. Bronstein, "Factors in Reduction of Infant Mortality in a Maternal and Infant Care Project," *Journal of the Medical Association of Georgia* 63 (1974): 425-29.

14. Minnesota Systems Research, "Children and Youth Projects," *Quarterly Summary Reports*, series 18 and 20 (April–June 1972 and October–December 1972).

15. J. Alpert et al., "Delivery of Health Care for Children: Report of an Experiment," *Pediatrics* 57 (1976): 917-31.

16. M. Klein et al., "The Impact of the Rochester Neighborhood Health Center on Hospitalization of Children, 1968-70," *Pediatrics* 51 (1973): 833-39.

17. L. Gordis, "Effectiveness of Comprehensive Care Programs in Preventing Rheumatic Fever," *New England Journal of Medicine* 289 (1973): 331-35.

18. J.W. Runyan, Jr., "The Memphis Chronic Disease Program: Comparisons in Outcome and the Nurse's Expanded Role," *Journal of the American Medical Association* 231 (1975): 164-67.

19. U.S. National Center for Health Statistics, *Monthly Vital Statistics Report Provisional Statistics Annual Summary for the United States*, 1976, vol. 25, no. 13, (Hyattsville, Md., December 12, 1977).

20. U.S. National Center for Health Statistics, *Monthly Vital Statistics Report*, *Final Mortality Statistics 1975*, vol. 25, no. 11, (Hyattsville, Md., February 11, 1977), table 12, p. 22; and U.S. National Center for Health Statistics, *Mortality Trends for Leading Causes of Death: United States 1950-69*, DHEW Publication No. (HRA) 74-1853, series 20, no. 16 (Rockville, Md., 1974).

CHAPTER 3

1. Marjorie S. Mueller and Robert M. Gibson, "National Health Expenditures Fiscal Year 1976," *Social Security Bulletin* 40, no. 4 (April 1977): 4-13.

2. "The Problem of Rising Health Care Costs," staff report, April 1976, Executive Office of the President, *Council on Wage and Price Stability* (Washington, D.C., 1976).

3. Theodore R. Marmor, "Rethinking National Health Insurance," *The Public Interest* 46 (Winter 1977): 73-95; Martin Feldstein, "The High Cost of Hospitals and What To Do About It," *The Public Interest* 48 (Summer 1977): 40-54; and Herbert E. Klarman, "The Financing of Health Care," *Daedalus* 106, no. 1 (Winter 1977): 215.

4. Bureau of the Census, *Persons Below Low Income Level and 125 Per Cent of Low Income Level in the Current Population Reports*, series p-60, nos. 68. 76, and 81 (Washington, D.C.: Government Printing Office, 1970).

5. Social Rehabilitation Service, *Public Assistance Recipients of Money Payments, States and Other Areas* (Washington, D.C.: Government Printing Office, 1971).

6. See Robert J. Blendon and Thomas W. Moloney, "Perspectives on the Growing Debate over the Cost of Medical Technologies" (paper delivered at the Sun Valley Forum, Sun Valley, Idaho, August 1977).

7. Personal Correspondence, Gordon L. McAndrew, superintendent of schools, Gary, Indiana.

8. National Council for Children and Youth, *America's Children, 1976: A bicentennial Assessment* (Washington, D.C., 1976), p. 15.

9. Institute of Medicine, *Assessment of Medical Care for Children* (Washington, D.C.: National Academy of Sciences, 1974), vol. 3, p. 2.

10. Philip R. Nader, "The Frequency and Nature of School Problems," in Robert J. Haggerty, Klaus J. Roghman, and Ivan B. Pless, eds., *Child Health and the Community* (New York: John Wiley & Sons, 1975), p. 101.

11. Institute of Medicine, *A Policy Statement: The Elderly and Functional Dependency* (Washington, D.C.: National Academy of Sciences, June 1977).

12. Karen Davis, "Health and the Great Society" (paper read before the Lyndon Baines Johnson Library Symposium, Austin, Texas, September 14, 1976), p. 24.

13. The Urban Institute, Office of Human Development, *Report of the Comprehensive Service Needs Study* (Washington, D.C.: Government Printing Office, 1975), p. 59.

14. David E. Rogers, "The Challenge of Primary Care," *Daedalus* 106, no. 1 (Winter 1977): 85.

15. David E. Rogers, "On Technologic Restraint," *Archives of Internal Medicine* 135 (October 1975): 1392-97.

CHAPTER 4

1. R.H. Egdahl et al., "The Potential of Organizations of Fee-for-Service Physicians for Achieving Significant Decreases in Hospitalization," *Annals of Surgery* 186, no. 3 (September 1977): 388-99; and Richard H. Egdahl and Diana Chapman Walsh, "Industry-Sponsored Health Programs: Basis for a New Hybrid Prepaid Plan," *The New England Journal of Medicine* 296, no. 23 (June 19, 1977): 1350-53.

2. American Medical Association, *Directory of Approved Internship and Residencies*, (Chicago: American Medical Association, 1967 and 1978).

3. "Face-off: Cost Containment vs. Chaos," *Patient Care*, January 1, 1977, p. 10.

4. Edmund G. Brown, Jr., "A Society of the People. And by. And for," *The New York Times*, June 6, 1977, p. 29.

5. Theodore R. Marmor, "Rethinking National Health Insurance," *The Public Interest* 46 (Winter 1977): 86-89.

6. Donald E. Pierson and Elizabeth H. Nicol, "The Fourth Year of The Brookline Early Education Project" (progress report prepared by the Brookline Early Education Project, Brookline, Massachusetts, January 1977).

7. See, for example, Michael H. Alderman and Ellie E. Schoenbaum, "Hypertension Control among Employed Persons in New York City: 1973-75," *Milbank Memorial Fund Quarterly* (Summer 1976): 367-77; Runyan, J.W., Jr., "The Memphis Chronic Disease Program," *Journal of the American Medical Association* 231, no. 3 (January 20, 1975): 264-67; and Thomas L. Petty, "Ambulatory Care for Emphysema and Chronic Bronchitis," *Chest* 58 (October 1970): 441-48.

PART II — INTRODUCTION

1. This is the opinion of others as well. See, for example, Derek C. Bok, *The President's Report: 1974 in 1975* (Cambridge, Mass.: Harvard University, 1975); and *Report of the Task Force on Regulation* (Albany: Hospital Association of New York State, 1976).

2. Johns Hopkins, Harvard, Yale, and Stanford lead a group of about a dozen medical schools that have said that they will forfeit federal capitation grants rather than comply with a provision of the Health Profession Education Assistance Act of 1976 that forces them to admit as juniors and seniors a government-set quota of foreign-trained Americans if they can meet considerably laxer admissions criteria than these schools normally require. See "Johns Hopkins Won't Accept U.S. Mandate," *The Baltimore Evening Sun*, August 15, 1977, pp. C1-C2; and "Four Medical Schools Draw the Line on Capitation," *Science*, September 9, 1977, p. 1066.

3. Walsh McDermott, "Medicine: The Public Good and One's Own," *Perspectives in Biology and Medicine* 21, no. 2 (Winter 1978): 167-87.

CHAPTER 5

1. C. Smythe, "Developing Medical Schools: An Interim Report," *Journal of Medical Education* 42, no. 11 (November 1967): 991-1004.
2. *American Hospital Association Annual Guide to the Health Care Field, 1976* ed. (Chicago: American Hospital Association, 1976).
3. Data derived from annual data of the National Center for Health Statistics and the American Hospital Association Annual Survey by Mr. John Craig, Health Policy Research Group, Georgetown University, Washington, D.C.
4. Walsh McDermott, Remarks at Medical Progress Dinner, the Waldorf Astoria, New York, December 7, 1961, published as "Science for the Individual—The University Medical Center," *Journal of Chronic Diseases* 16 (1963): 105-10.

CHAPTER 6

1. *1977-78 Directory of American Medical Education* (Washington, D.C.: Association of American Medical Colleges, 1977), pp. vi-ix; and *United States Department of Commerce News*, April 14, 1977, pp. 1-4.
2. M. Alfred Haynes and Michael R. McGarvey, "Physicians, Hospitals, and Patients in the Inner City," in John C. Norman, ed., *Medicine in the Ghetto* (New York: Appleton-Century-Croft, 1969), p. 117.
3. *United States Statistical Abstract 1976* (Washington, D.C.: Government Printing Office, 1977), Tables 21, 23.
4. Morton Grodzins, *The Metropolitan Area as a Racial Problem* (Pittsburgh: University of Pittsburgh Press, 1958), p. 3.
5. John H. Strange, "Racial Segregation in the Metropolis," in Michael N. Danielson, ed., *Metropolitan Politics: A Reader* (Boston: Little, Brown & Co., 1966), p. 43.
6. See Marvin R. Weisbord, "Why Organization Development Hasn't Worked (So Far) in Medical Centers," *Health Care Management Review* (Spring 1976), pp. 17-28.
7. *NIH Factbook* (Chicago: Marquis Academic Media, 1976), pp. 109-11.
8. "Medical Education in the United States, 1962-1963." *Journal of the American Medical Association*, 186(7), November 16, 1963, Chicago, 1963; and "Medical Education in the United States, 1975-1976." *Journal of the American Medical Association*, 236(26), December 27, 1976, Chicago, 1976.
9. Data supplied by Mr. Charles R. Buck, Jr., director of planning, The Johns Hopkins Medical Institutions, Baltimore, Maryland.
10. *American Hospital Association Guide to the Health Care Field*, 1955 and 1975 eds. (Chicago: American Hospital Association, 1955 and 1975).
11. Martin S. Feldstein, *The Rising Cost of Hospital Care* (Washington, D.C.: Information Resources Press, 1971), Table 5.6.

12. Data supplied by Mr. Charles R. Buck, Jr., director of planning, The Johns Hopkins Medical Institutions, Baltimore, Maryland.

13. *Report of the Task Force on Regulation* (Albany: Hospital Association of New York State, 1976).

14. Public Law 89–97, Section 102A, passed July 30, 1965.

15. Karen, David, "Economic Theories of Behavior in Nonprofit, Private Hospitals," Brookings Reprint 239 (Washington, D.C.: The Brookings Institution), Table 1, 1972.

16. Marjorie S. Mueller and Robert M. Gibson, "National Health Expenditures Fiscal Year 1975," *Social Security Bulletin* 39, no. 2 (February 1976).

17. U.S. Department of Commerce, Bureau of Census, *Statistical Abstracts of the United States 1976* (Washington, D.C., 1976), Table 1309; and U.S. Department of Labor, Bureau of Labor Statistics, Employment and Earnings March 1976, vol. 22, no. 9, (Washington, D.C., 1976) Table B–2; and *American Hospital Association Guide to the Health Care Field*, 1976 ed.; (Chicago: American Hospital Association, 1976); and U.S. Department of Commerce, Bureau of Census, *County Business Patterns 1973* (Washington, D.C., December 1975), CBP 73–1.

18. Kerr L. White, T. Franklin Williams, and Bernard G. Greenberg, "The Ecology of Medical Care," *New England Journal of Medicine* 255 (November 2, 1961): 885–92.

19. Data supplied by Mr. Charles R. Buck, Jr., director of planning, The Johns Hopkins Medical Institutions, Baltimore, Maryland.

20. Renee Fox, "The Medicalization and Demedicalization of American Society," *Daedalus* (Winter 1977): 9–22.

21. Anthony J. Reading and Torrey C. Brown, "Interdisciplinary Alcoholism Education for Medical and Paramedical Personnel," *Maryland State Medical Journal* 20 (March 1971): 85.

CHAPTER 7

1. Harlan Cleveland, "How Do You Get Everyone in on the Act and Still Get Some Action?" *Educational Record* 55, no. 3 (Summer 1974).

2. David E. Rogers, "Reflections on a Medical School Deanship," *The Pharos of Alpha Omega Alpha* 38, no. 3 (July 1975): 115–21.

3. Marvin R. Weisbord, "Why Organization Development Hasn't Worked (So Far) in Medical Centers," *Health Care Management Review* (Spring 1976), p. 19.

4. David E. Rogers, "Preparing for a Balanced State Society," *The Pharos of Alpha Omega Alpha* 39, no. 4 (October 1976): 136–38.

5. M.T. MacEachern, *Hospital Organization and Management* (Berwyn, Ill.: Physicians' Record Company, 1962), p. 21.

6. Institute of Medicine. *Controlling the Supply of Hospital Beds* (Washington, D.C.: National Academy of Sciences, 1976).

7. Robert J. Blendon, "The Reform of Ambulatory Care: A Financial Paradox" *Medical Care*, vol. 14, no. 6 (June 1976): 526–34.

8. Walsh McDermott, "Sciences for the Individual—The University Medical Center," *Journal of Chronic Diseases*, vol. 16 (1963): 105–110.

PART III – INTRODUCTION

1. Walsh McDermott, "General Medical Care: Identification and Analysis of Alternative Approaches," *The Johns Hopkins Medical Journal* 135, no. 5 (November 1974): 293.

CHAPTER 8

1. *Journal of the American Medical Association*, 238 (26) (Chicago: American Medical Association, December 1977).

2. Daniel H. Funkenstein, "Medical Students, Medical Schools, and Society During Three Eras," in R.H. Combes and C.E. Vincent, eds., *Psychosocial Aspects of Medical Training* (Springfield, Ill.: Charles C. Thomas, Publisher, 1971).

3. See William G. Bowen, "Admissions and the Relevance of Race," *Princeton Alumni Weekly*, September 26, 1977, pp. 7-13; and McGeorge Bundy, "The Issue Before the Court: Who Gets Ahead in America?" *Atlantic* 240 (November 1977): 41-50.

CHAPTER 9

1. Rene Dubos, *Louis Pasteur: Free Lance of Science* (Boston: Little, Brown & Company, 1950), p. 383.

2. E. Grey Dimond, "Courage Beyond Science" (commencement address at the Hahnemann Graduate School and Medical College, Philadelphia, June 3, 1976; reprinted in *Vesper Exchange* 34 (Spring 1977).

3. Clifton Meador, "Symptons of Unknown Origin: Suggested Classification and Principles of Management" (Nashville: Vanderbilt University School of Medicine, forthcoming).

4. I have expressed my views on this in greater detail elsewhere. See David E. Rogers, "Presidential Address on Technologic Restraint," *Transaction of the Association of American Physicians* 88 (1975).

5. Quoted in George L. Engel, "The Care of the Patient: Art or Science," *The Johns Hopkins Medical Journal* 140, no. 5 (May 1977): 222.

6. Daniel H. Funkenstein, "The Changing Pool of Medical School Applicants," *Harvard Medical Alumni Bulletin* (Summer 1967).

7. Harrison G. Gough and Wallace B. Hall, "A Prospective Study of Personality Changes in Students in Medicine, Dentistry, and Nursing," *Research in Higher Education* 1 (1973): 138.

8. Harrison G. Gough, "What Happens to Creative Medical Students?" *Journal of Medical Education* 51 (June 1976): 461-67; and Harrison G. Gough, "Some Predictive Implications of Premedical Scientific Competence and Preferences, *Journal of Medical Education* 53 (April 1978): 291-99.

CHAPTER 10

1. Much has been written on the potential overproduction of physicians in the United States. For two recent expositions of the problem, see the Carnegie

Council on Policy Studies in Higher Education, *Progress and Problems in Medical and Dental Education: Federal Support Versus Federal Control* (San Francisco: Jossey—Bass, Inc., Publishers, 1976), pp. 3 8-9, 32; and U.S. Department of Health, Education, and Welfare, *The Supply of Health Manpower: 1970 Profiles and Projections to 1990*, DHEW Publication No. (HRA) 75-38 (Washington, D.C.: Government Printing Office, 1974), pp. 53-55.

2. See David E. Rogers, "Point of View," *HOPMED*, no. 14 (January 1972).

3. Personal communication, Michael A. Simpson, Department of Psychiatry, and J.F. Mustard, M.D., dean, Health Sciences, McMaster University, Hamilton, Ontario, Canada.

4. David E. Rogers, "The Doctor Himself Must Become the Treatment," *The Pharos of Alpha Omega Alpha* 37, no. 4 (October 1974): 126.

5. Jeremiah A. Barondess, "Science in Medicine: Some Negative Feedbacks," *Archives of Internal Medicine* 134, no. 1 (January 1974): 152.

6. George L. Engel, "The Care of the Patient: Art of Science," *The Johns Hopkins Medical Journal* 1401, no. 5 (May 1977): 222.

7. Richard Fletcher, "Sociological Observations of the Holistic Health Movement," in Donnie J. Self, ed., *Social Issues in Health Care* (Norfolk, Va.: Teagle & Little, 1977), pp. 90-100.

Index

About the Author

David E. Rogers is the physician-president of The Robert Wood Johnson Foundation, a philanthropy devoting its resources to bettering the health and medical care of Americans. From 1968 to 1972, he served as the Dean of the Medical Faculties and Vice President (Medicine) of the Johns Hopkins University, a position he accepted after 10 years as Professor and Chairman of the Department of Medicine at Vanderbilt University. Dr. Rogers is an editor of the *Year Book of Medicine* and the author of numerous papers in the field of infectious disease, medical education, and American health and medical care.

2/11